The Hypochondriac's Handbook

The Hypochondriac's Handbook

DR LEE SCHREINER & DR GEORGE THOMAS

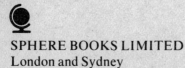

SPHERE BOOKS LIMITED
London and Sydney

First published in Great Britain by
Enigma Books 1983
Copyright © 1983 Dr Lee Schreiner and Dr George Thomas
Published by Sphere Books Ltd 1984
30-32 Gray's Inn Road, London WC1X 8JL

TRADE
MARK

Set in Melior

Printed and bound in Great Britain by
Cox & Wyman Ltd, Reading

Contents

Introduction

The right to dissemble; to speak freely of your symptoms without restraint; to bare arms or for that matter anything else to the doctor of your choice at the hour of your choice – thus would Magna Carta have enshrined your rights as a patient if our forefathers hadn't been off nursing their lumbago with leeches. After all, good health has always been an Englishman's inalienable right. In a society where happiness could truly be pursued and eventually cornered, medical care would be readily available to all who wanted it, without costing them their savings or dignity.

As we all know, however, medicine falls far short of this lofty ideal. Casualty departments do not have welcome mats nor do they promote a Happy Hour. Hospitals don't offer away-day breaks.[1] There are no laws forbidding doctors from rolling their eyes. Instead we have a health service that cruelly provides intensive care to the patient only when he needs it. When finally he starts getting the attention he's been seeking, he's too sick to enjoy it.

One reason is that there just aren't enough doctors to go around. There are fewer than 25,000 physicians in the U.K., and at any given time about a quarter of them are tied up working on their cross-court passing shots. Another twenty percent are busy applying for grants. Many of the rest are psychiatrists, who may just be making matters worse.

Competing for the attention of these doctors are over

---

1. Although one can occasionally arrange a cruise-to-nowhere.

fifty-five million prospective patients. Of these, about five hundred and seventeen are perfectly healthy, and live in Devonshire. They need not be counted in calculations of how medical care is made available. Many others who are genuinely ill are poor, can't speak English, or don't know anybody, and thus have difficulty in obtaining medical attention. They don't count either. Still, there have always been lots of people who are covered by neither category trying to elbow their way into the waiting room.

The forgotten victims of this crush are the hypochondriacs. These gentle souls harm no one, and never asked for much – just reassurance, understanding and their doctors' home phone numbers. In less turbulent times, they were respected members of the community who were prized for their ability to identify poisonous plants. Gradually, though, these patients have come to feel that they are not welcome. Little things added up. No more free pills, for example. Some noted that most patients were encouraged to undress almost immediately, while they were not even allowed to unbutton their overcoats. Others found it significant that before they were shown into the doctor's office, he had all the chairs removed. Eventually, they were forced into a hypochondriac's underground, subsisting on Beecham's powders, vitamin C, and home health encyclopedias.

Recently, though, doctors have noted a new militancy among these patients. They're tired of scorn; they will no longer tolerate condescension. They argue convincingly that hypochondriasis is not a disease, though almost everything else is. 'Pills, not ill will' is their motto. They've stepped out of the medicine closet and into the emergency ward.

Sociologists are hardly surprised, for in so many ways the Hypochondriac Movement is a logical outcome of the Me Decade. It is the final preoccupation with the self – flavoured by the assumption that the self is sick, or at least headed in that general direction.

Technology can achieve much, but irresistible forces are irresistible forces. In the end, these patients know, is the end. They don't need to ask death, 'Where is thy sting?' They know where it is. Right behind them and gaining fast.

The Hypochondriac's Handbook is both a manifesto for this movement and a naked attempt to cash in on it. The book itself was inspired by fervent requests from patients for more and more information. They would bring us a common complaint, and want to know the worst possible disease that it could represent. We gave them simple, unambiguous answers in terms that they could understand.

Their tears of gratitude moved us. Eventually, though, performing this service of compassion became tedious even after we added dance steps and made them beat time with a reflex hammer. Thus we began to circulate mimeographed sheets simply listing the most popular complaints, along with our estimate of how much time the sufferer might have left if things went badly. (e.g. 'Runny nose – three months.')

The thirst for information was endless. Soon patients were not satisfied with the mundane. They wanted the lowdown on the rarest syndromes with the most innocuous initial symptoms – diseases they were better off not knowing about. They requested details of infections they could catch from their pets, or wanted information about how exercise can take years off their lives and render miserable the time left to them. They wanted to know how to recognise their own psychiatric emergencies, how to examine themselves when no one else would and how to get into hospital when they felt lonely. They didn't want to know about the possibility of dying from an allergic reaction during sex, but we told them anyway.

Thus The Hypochondriac's Handbook became what it is – a handbook for hypochondriacs. It is the fruit of our loom, a general guide by which to live, full of the medical background you need to manipulate your doctor and loved ones. Every disease described is real. No punches are pulled. No data is falsified. All of the studies mentioned and pieces of medical information presented are absolutely true, though a lot of it is twisted and taken out of context.

This book will teach you about dozens of diseases that you almost certainly do not have. Still, they have been carefully chosen so that your doctor will have a hell of a time ruling them out once you have raised the possibility. He will be forced to put you through an extensive evaluation which might well entail admission into hospital. If the results are entirely negative, the chances that you have some other fatal disease are slightly reduced. Of course, the tests themselves might bump you off.

Needless to say, these tests will be expensive which raises the question of how far you should go in abusing the National Health Service. The sad fact is that we live in a time of diminishing resources and increasing needs. You should make every attempt to ignore this bad news. Endless worrying about how society is going to pay for your stomach X-rays is only going to upset your stomach. You must consider the health service a precious resource, like our national parks, and visit it as often as possible.

It has been written that the road to bad health is paved with good intentions. With the purchase of this book, you have made the first, faltering move. Now, if you'll just follow us, we'll guide you the rest of the way.

1
Ten diseases you were better off not knowing about

Few tasks in a doctor's life are as emotionally trying as telling a patient who is convinced he is ill that nothing is wrong. The ensuing hostilities can be brutal; but then no one ever promised that medicine would be pretty. Most doctors eventually learn how to handle the common, everyday hypochondriac – the twenty-two year old man with a 'heart attack', for example or the middle aged woman with prostate trouble. These patients are examined, carefully reassured, and then served a restraining order if they refuse to leave the surgery.

By contrast, we doctors live in fear of the medically sophisticated hypochondriac who may arrive on a stretcher complaining about a disease we have never heard of. These patients become neurotically obsessed with exceedingly rare diseases partly because their chances of actually having what they are worried about are considerably reduced, but also because a good deal of time and effort will be expended before the disease can be ruled out.

A doctor can look at a chest X-ray and be fairly sure within seconds that you don't have lung cancer. But try telling him that you have *bangungut*, also known as 'Nightmare Syndrome' (victims go to bed, thrash, cough, and cannot be resuscitated) because your father, grandfather, and two brothers all died of it — then pass out in his office.

He will be quite careful before dismissing you as a fake. If you're lucky, the subsequent treatment may involve so many examinations and tests that a real disease might turn up before it gets too much of a hold.

Not surprisingly, doctors try to keep the lay public from finding out about these really weird diseases. It's perfectly okay for a TV soap opera to raise consciousness about jogger's knee, but no doctor will ever advise on a script about Familial Periodic Paralysis. The working theory is that an ounce of prevention is worth a pound of cure, and what they don't know won't hurt them.

Throughout our careers we have agreed with this philosophy and honoured the vow of secrecy. But the pleas of patients starved for inside information have touched us. In addition, we've been offered a lot of money. Thus, we present ten diseases that you were definitely better off not knowing about.

Most of these syndromes will make it difficult for those afflicted to find flat-mates, but they'll have no problem finding a seat on a crowded bus.

All have three features in common:

They are rare.

They are real.

They begin with innocuous everyday symptoms.

Orzechowski's Syndrome

When Orzechowski's Syndrome was first described in 1913, theologians could have taken this rare disorder as proof that God loves a good Polish joke. After all, why else would He create such a ridiculous disease as an afterthought to the common cold. Parliament may pass legislation this way, but He ought to know better.

This disease actually begins with a viral illness indistinguishable from an ordinary head cold. After a few days, the 'cold' clears up, and the virus appears beaten. Rommel often used this same tactic to great effect in North Africa during World War II.

A few days, later, however, the virus returns for an encore. You develop a headache and a fever and from there it's all downhill. Your day becomes punctuated by sudden attacks in which your eyeballs start to flutter abruptly from side-to-side. The mildest of visual stimuli set off these spells. Simply shifting your gaze or blinking can trigger several attacks a day, each lasting minutes to hours. Crossing your eyes is really asking for it. The result is chaos for your vision, unless you are driving in Paris where it may actually help.

Fortunately, those you meet may not notice your eyes. They will be too busy staring at the rest of your body, which will be providing a visual explanation of how Orzechowski's Syndrome got its nickname: Dancing Hands, Dancing Feet syndrome. During these spells, torsos twitch and limbs flail, as if responding to some primaeval rhythm. Sitting next to Orzechowski patients on tube-trains can be a brutal experience. It's usually safest to simply hand over your wallet without trying to resist.

The mere sight of a patient with Orzechowski's Syndrome makes children cry and dogs howl but, oddly enough, the victims themselves are almost indifferent. This is probably due to the viral inflammation of the brain. Orzechowski himself noted that most sufferers do not seem to be bothered by their rather absurd appearance, and cited that as useful in making the diagnosis.

The rest of the world feels quite differently, however. The symptoms almost always disappear within a few weeks but by that time you will have been dropped by your entire social circle. We tell patients who are upset about the effect they create to move to

London for the duration of their illness so as to be less conspicuous. They can rent a small room in Notting Hill and spend their days mingling with the crowds at Madame Tussaud's or the Houses of Parliament until respectable society is ready to take them back.

Ascher's Syndrome

Ascher's Syndrome – perhaps better known as Double Lip Disease – was first described by the German physician K. W. Ascher in 1920 in an article called 'Blepharochalasia mit Struma und Doppellippe'. This disease remains a mystery to most physicians, who are still waiting for the film version. Nevertheless, experts see Ascher's as the best chance most people have of looking like a film-star. Unfortunately, the star in question is Charles Laughton.

Ascher's starts with a little swelling around the eyes and lips – nothing new to survivors of boxing matches and stag parties. This puffiness, however, is caused by lymphocytes – white blood cells that ordinarily are key parts of your body's defence against infections. For reasons known only to themselves, thousands of these cells turn on the patient and start migrating from the blood to the eyes and lips for the express purpose of destroying all the elastic fibres – the little strands that provide shape and resilience to your face. Lose them, and you lose forever the chance to model for *Vogue*.

As they are attacked, the lips and gums become inflamed, swell to several times their original size, and finally give the appearance of double or triple lips. At this point, whistling will produce a resounding raspberry and you may have to give up your trumpet lessons. Next, the tissue around the eyes becomes so loose and baggy that your eyes slide down into your cheeks. Eventually, your face resembles an Albanian village in a mudslide.

Partly because all lab tests are normal in Ascher's

Syndrome, and partly because there is no cure, doctors tend to delay before making the correct diagnosis. They will argue that your parents looked that way *too* when they were your age. Do not be stalled by such tactics. At the first sign of sag, find yourself a good plastic surgeon.

Familial Periodic Paralysis

Familial periodic paralysis is one of those rare disorders in which the name actually conveys meaningful information about the disease instead of the doctors who discovered it. Medical historians cannot completely explain this phenomenon, but apparently the illness was recognized around the turn of the century – after the birth of neurology as a speciality, but before neurologists fully understood the art of self-promotion.

This disease, as advertised, runs in families and is characterised by recurrent episodes in which the patient simply cannot move. Of course, there are plenty of exceptions. Some victims have no recognisable family history; others never have a second attack because, well, they don't do so well during the first.

The typical patient is under thirty when he has his initial spell, and lives out a normal lifespan – although much of it is spent horizontally. The attacks begin with a sense of heaviness in the legs. This heaviness soon gives way to genuine weakness, which ascends inch by inch. In a surprisingly short time, victims find themselves completely paralyzed from the neck down. The weakness peaks in about an hour and clears over a day. The brain itself is unaffected, so as you lie on the beach and watch the tide come in, you'll have plenty of time to worry about the decline of liberalism.

Abortive attacks, consisting of stiffness and a reluctance to move, can be the first sign of illness. Precocious children often cite this disease as an explanation of why they cannot answer their mothers while watching TV.

To ascertain which children are lying and to detect impending attacks of your own, we urge you to recognize the 'prodrome' or warning signs that precede spells. Excessive thirst or hunger, sleepiness, irritability, or sweatiness can all presage an attack. Any of these tip-offs will send some of our regular patients to bed until the danger period has passed, whether they have the disease or not.

Exactly what causes this paralysis is not clear, though some biochemical disturbance seems involved. Most patients improve with potassium supplements, but beyond that, doctors can only advise avoiding the precipitating factors described by other victims. The most common of these are alcohol, excitement, exposure to cold, and menstruation. Given this warning, doctors feel, further attacks are the patient's fault.

Ondine's Curse

Ondine: Live Hans. You too will forget.

Hans: Live! It's easy to say. If at least I could work up a little interest in living, but I'm too tired to make the effort. Since you left me, Ondine, all the things my body once did by itself, it does now only by special order ... It's an exhausting piece of management I've undertaken. I have to supervise five senses, two hundred bones, a thousand muscles. A single moment of inattention and I forget to breathe. He died, they will say, because it was a nuisance to breathe ...

From Act III, *Ondine* by Jean Giraudoux

Long before *Dallas*, long before Lucretia Borgia, there was Ondine – a sea nymph from early German mythology who could have taught Charles Bronson a thing or two about getting even. She loved, and was then betrayed by, her mortal husband – a knight named Hans. The punishment for his infidelity was severe – Ondine took all automatic bodily functions from him. When her lover finally fell asleep, it was for keeps.

Fantasy, right? Well, take a deep breath, (Inhale) try to imagine how Hans felt and read on. (Exhale). Sometimes, expiration imitates art.

In 1956 (Inhale) three patients turned up in San Francisco with a strange problem, even for California. (Exhale). All three breathed normally on command. (Inhale) but, like Hans, if not reminded, they forgot to breathe. (Exhale). In each case (Inhale) difficulties had developed slowly after normal youths. (Exhale). Two had seizures while they slept (Inhale) because of an oxygen deficiency. (Exhale). By the time they consulted doctors (Inhale) they needed respirators to assist their breathing every night. (Exhale). Since then (Inhale) more than forty similar cases have been found, and the syndrome has been called 'Ondine's Curse.' (Exhale). Patients are twenty to sixty-five years old (Inhale) and first complain of headaches, shortness of breath, and decreased endurance. (Exhale). In several cases (Inhale) autopsies showed damage of unknown cause to the brain's breathing centre. (Exhale).

Fortunately (Inhale) severe cases of Ondine's Curse are rare. (Exhale). In fact (Inhale) doctors consider the disease's main danger the chance that people will read about it (Exhale) become very conscious of their breathing (Inhale) and panic (Inhale) because they aren't sure (Inhale) that they will be able to breathe (Inhale) if they stop thinking about it. (INHALE).

Lassa Fever

Among the worries unique to our times, we can definitely include Lassa Fever. In the good old days, this virus was confined to West Africa, where no one went except by accident. Now it can pop up anywhere, thanks to air travel. And when it does, doctors agree, it's bad.

How bad is Lassa Fever? It is so bad it makes spending one's entire life in Bognor Regis look good. It is worse than detergent commercials. It is one of the most lethal and contagious diseases known to man. It is so bad that if you walk into a doctor's office and tell him that you have Lassa Fever, he will not touch you, come close, or brother you in any way while you rifle the medicine cabinet or play with his stethoscope. Such is the fear aroused by Lassa Fever since its discovery a decade ago. Ironically, it begins like most other viral syndromes, with fever, malaise, muscle aches, and a sore throat. Similarity to a cold ends there, however, as the virus then moves through the entire body and persuades virtually every organ to close shop. The virus is known for two distinguishing features – a high mortality rate and a startling ability to spread from one person to another.

Take, for example, the first described outbreak of Lassa Fever. Four experts in infectious diseases were studying viral infections in West African missionaries in 1969 when they heard of the case of 'L. W.' an elderly nurse working in a missionary hospital in the remote town of Lassa, located in the Cameroon foothills of Nigeria. Death comes easily to the anonymous poor in that region. Often, they have so many diseases that figuring out which is killing them is academic. But it is a safe bet that one of the last patients cared for by L. W. was dying of Lassa Fever, and that he gave the virus to her.

On January 12, 1969, she complained of a backache. The next day she developed a sore throat; on the following day she was unable to swallow. Unresponsive to antibiotics, she was flown in desperation to a larger hospital in Jos, Nigeria, on January 25. She died the next day.

The nurse on duty when she arrived that night in Jos, a forty-five year-old woman whom we shall call 'C. S.', saw that her new patient was choking on her own secretions. Wrapping her finger in gauze, C. S. reached in and cleared them away. Later she realised that she had a small cut on her finger. She washed it and applied antiseptics, but it was too late.

On February 3, she developed a backache and a sore throat, and then a fever and a headache. In eleven days she too was dead.

A third nurse, 'L. P.', cared for the dying night nurse and assisted at her autopsy. On February 20, she noted a mild fever as she left work. By February 23, she had a sore throat and laboratory findings suggested that she had become the latest victim of this new disease. Unnerved, the doctors in Jos packed the patient off for the Presbyterian Hospital in New York City, the nearest good hospital.

News of her impending admission inspired many of the staff physicians to volunteer for tours of duty in Vietnam, which has no direct bus service from Nigeria. When she arrived in New York, the nurse with Lassa Fever was immediately placed in full isolation – the medical equivalent of cling film – to protect those who tended her around the clock. Despite running temperatures as high as 107°, she survived, although rumour has it that someone grabbed her handbag. Her recovery took months.

Meanwhile, Lassa Fever maintained its dance of death. One of the researchers travelled to Nigeria to study the cases that continued to turn up. On February 18, 1970, four weeks after her paper describing the outbreak was accepted for publication, she died of Lassa Fever in Jos, the first outbreak's final victim.

Needless to say, this epidemic created quite a stir in the medical community. For years, many nervous doctors considered the disease so dangerous that they refused to say its name out loud, or move their lips while reading about it. A few extremists continue to examine patients with backaches only if they wear a paper bag over their heads. The only positive aspect about all this is that it's pretty easy to book hotel rooms in Lassa on short notice; and if they do happen to be full, vacancies usually develop by the time you arrive.

Fortunately, most of you have almost no chance of catching Lassa Fever as long as you do not live within a hundred miles of a city with an international airport.

Steel – Richardson – Olsewski Syndrome

Steel–Richardson–Olszewski Syndrome (SRO) is one of a large number of degenerative neurological disorders to which a simple diagnostic test can be applied – if you can remember the name and spell it correctly without peeking, then you probably don't have the disease.

Like most of these syndromes, SRO begins in middle age or later and then progresses relentlessly as the brain is replaced by packing material. Victims eventually become demented, move with great reluctance and unsteadiness, and have difficulty speaking clearly. Unless you are a high court judge, these problems usually force an early retirement.

SRO is especially unique for its initial symptom, the inability to look down – an unbearable deficiency for residents of Knightsbridge. Early on, victims of this disease lose strength in the muscles that turn the eyeballs downwards. This deficiency progresses slowly at first and may not be immediately noticed. Only in retrospect does the patient remember that the first ominous sign was tripping on a curb. Or stumbling on the stairs. Or spilling food on his tie. Eventually, the body becomes inflexible and the soul applies for a transfer. Complications set in and everyone calls it a day.

Now, no one is saying you have SRO just because a few peas rolled off your fork at dinner tonight. Then

10

again, no one is saying you don't. It's just too soon to tell.

The Cinderella Syndrome

There's more than one Cinderella Syndrome in medicine, and none involves Koo Stark. The oddest is a skin condition known as erythema dyschromicum perstans, which may not help you meet a prince, but could get you into the Sunday papers. After all, how many people have skin that makes them walking Rorschach tests?

This rare disease begins as a small grey patch the hue of burnt newspaper under the eyes or on the arms. The spot enlarges into an irregular ring as other patches, in varying shades of grey, pop up elsewhere. These blotches shift around and merge with each other, forming bizarre patterns. It's a bit like having a movie-map showing the growth of the Third Reich projected on your chest, only this time Germany wins.

The patches are caused by your own white blood cells, the body's soldiers that are ordinarily assigned the job of gobbling up invading bacteria. In patients suffering from the Cinderella Syndrome, however, the white cells act like sailors on leave after six months at sea. They abandon the blood vessels and roar into the skin where they eat melanin, the pigment granules that give skin its colour.

Having done one foolish thing, the engorged, gaily-hued cells don't know what to do next, so they wander aimlessly under the skin creating wavy lines as they move. These migrations offer one small hope to victims – if they don't like the way they look one week, there's always the chance they'll be happier the next.

The rash doesn't respond to any known treatment, though sometimes it disappears on its own when white blood cells decide to face the music and go home. Until then, patients must put up with the good and bad results of having shifting ink blots on their faces and bodies. On one hand, previously affectionate people turn on you as your mottled visage begins to remind them of some primal childhood terror. On the other, you'll never have trouble getting into discos again.

Lethal Midline Granuloma

Lethal Midline Granuloma is a rare inflammatory disease of unexplained nature that is every bit as bad as it sounds – maybe worse. It is so unpleasant that we'd rather not go into details other than to warn you that the first symptoms are a runny nose or sinus conditions. As for what happens after that, let's just say that it is a good idea to check that the damage isn't really due to tuberculosis, leprosy, or end-stage syphilis – all diseases that you'd rather have than lethal midline granuloma.

Beyond that, we just don't feel like discussing it, okay?

Cobalt Beer Syndrome

Picture the scene . . . It's the end of another long day of punching cows. A herd of horses with tall men on them stampede the local saloon. The next shot shows one or two cowpokes inside, exchanging admiring glances with a beer-bearing beauty.

Where are the other cowboys? If they're regulars at the saloon, they could have cobalt beer syndrome, in which case it's going to take them a long time to get from the corral to the bar. With swollen legs and decaying hearts, just getting out of the saddle could take up most of the Happy Hour.

The syndrome was born over twenty years ago, when beer manufacturers discovered that cobalt enhanced the flavour of their product. Some brewers began to add cobalt in liberal doses to their special brews. The result was a quick victory for free enterprise in its periodic range wars with public health.

After several years of dedicated boozing, the cobalt settles in the heart – where the muscle fibres swell and die. As the heart weakens, blood backs up in the veins like water behind a damn. The increased pressure causes swelling first of the legs, then of the belly and scrotum. (This process explains the distinctive walk of many cowboys.)

Poor oxygen uptake by the slowly circulating blood turns the cowboy a dusky blue. He also becomes kind of slow talkin', because not so much blood gets uphill to his brain anymore. What does is full of junk usually cleaned up by his liver, which is also in the process of checking out for the last roundup.

Doctors only recognized this syndrome in the 1960s and, eventually, beer manufacturers were persuaded to take the cobalt out of their secret formulas. Still, cobalt is an occasional pollutant in the water used to make beer and God knows what they've added to take its place.

Prader Willi Syndrome

The insight that human beings are irrational creatures is often illuminated by the dim glow of a refrigerator's light between one and two a.m. on a Saturday night. Bored and a little drunk, you survey all that is cool and green, and you wonder – 'What shall I eat?'

Inexorably, the question becomes, 'Why do I eat?' You go through the motions of rational discourse. You eat because you are starved for love, because you are hungry for spiritual nourishment, because that girl went to Rome and never came back. All this thinking only makes you hungrier. You pop some lasagne in the oven and you open another beer.

An hour later, the radio disc-jockey has signed off

and the lasagne is gone. Only the top got warm. You lie in bed, in that expanding trough in your mattress, understanding that you've done it again. You've eaten too much – far more than you wanted. Your pyjamas feel tight and you have trouble getting comfortable. The bedspread seems heavier than you remember and you're vaguely short of breath. Your stomach blocks the view to your feet, and your chin blocks the view to your stomach. You feel fat. Fat, fat, fat.

In the final analysis, there are only two possible explanations for your sudden identification with beached whales. Some earn fatness; others have it thrust upon them. If your idea of a double date is to take fish and chips to the cinema, you are in the former category, where most people reside. If you eat the fish and chips, the greaseproof-bags and the newspaper however, you may be one of the guiltless inhabitants of the second. You may have Prader Willi Syndrome.

The bearers of this uncommon, inherited disorder are *really* fat. Some unknown neurological defect drives them to eat – any time, any place, anything. For them, it's one a.m. Saturday night all year long and the entire world, with all its riches, is a big refrigerator.

The Prader Willi literature is full of stories of one-man supermarket sweeps. For example, one child regularly ate several loaves of bread directly from the freezer, or two entire cakes at a sitting. By the age of five, he had already had his stomach pumped many times at hospitals after swallowing a variety of noxious substances including DDT, fruit stones and detergents.

Some victims have been caught stealing food, rifling dustbins and eating animal food after chasing their pets away. Others have been known to eat entire jars of mayonnaise or packets of butter. One boy helped his class bake a dozen apple pies as a school project. During the afternoon break, he sneaked back in and consumed eight of them.

Most Prader Willi victims are a little slow in intelligence tests. They also tend to be short, and to have poor muscle tone and underdeveloped genitals. What separates them from the rest of us is that they are almost always extraordinarily pleasant people.

That these diseases exist at all demands reflection on the nature of the universe and our place in it. You could conclude that any system that can come up with syndromes like these has no ultimate purpose; that life, as Hobbes put it, is nasty, British, and short. Conversely, you may reason that the existence of such bizarre disorders stands as proof that there is a higher order of Intelligence, a Supreme Being with an ultimate plan to which we are not privy. We would agree, though we would add that if a Divine Providence truly created these diseases, He is not only pretty clever but also really pissed off.

2
Common complaints and the worst possible diseases they could represent

Ever since Man first discovered his own mortality, he has been seeing it behind every rock, tree and bush. Naturally, this insight changed the way he looked at the world and his all-too-precarious place in it. Man did not become less contemplative – he merely started contemplating different things; sores that were slow to heal, for example, or subtle changes in bowel and bladder habits. The meaning of life suddenly seemed less pressing an issue than the question of how to prolong it. The intense desire to understand one's role in a universe supervised by unseen and powerful gods became secondary to the intense desire to understand what in hell was causing that red, itchy rash between the toes.

Before doctors were created, Man sought to master these bodily complaints through religion. Indeed, some believe that the word 'symptom' is derived from a Greek phrase meaning. 'My throat is sore; call the priest.' Patients tried various rituals to fend off the aches and pains of life in the ancient world. Smearing

17

mud in one's hair, solemn chanting, and eating an apple a day all seemed promising at first, but eventually proved false hopes. Once people found that no church had a prayer for irregularity, they gave up on religion altogether.

At first, medicine could do no better. In ancient cultures doctors did not understand the physiology behind diseases any more than did priests. They were full of purpose, but short on power – and had little to offer or even do. As far as we can tell, physicians in early Greece had no day-to-day function other than concocting suicide potions and practising long putts in a special area of the temple.

Chinese physicians were the first to try to pick up early signs of impending doom – though not by choice. A certain emperor decided that paying doctors when ill made little sense. It seemed more logical to pay the physician only when one was feeling well. When the emperor himself felt poorly, he made his court physicians feel even worse. He put them to death.

The court physicians, a group naturally prone to nervousness, took to dropping in on the emperor every day just to see how things were going. Legend has it that a few of the younger doctors, lately graduated from Chinese medical school, began calling on him every thirty minutes until the emperor had two of them put away for breathing too heavily on his feet.

Since that shaky start, doctors have learned a great deal about symptoms and their implications. Patients, too, have discovered the importance of keeping up with the latest insights into the body's imperative to reproduce and deteriorate, though not necessarily in that order. Thus, today, everyone knows that if your tongue is too smooth you could have pernicious anemia causing low blood counts and dementia; that bad breath can mean gangrene of the stomach; or that insomnia may mean cirrhosis of the liver.

Instead of such routine fare, this chapter will focus on some common complaints and the worst possible

18

diseases they could represent. The worried patient need no longer be afraid to present his blemish or discharge to the modern doctor, only to have his concern scorned as a groundless fear. This chapter will put some solid ground under your fears. Now, instead of asking the doctor what *he* thinks of that symptom you have been observing – and perhaps nursing when it threatened to falter – you can tell the doctor what *you* think of it. The two of you will get on as never before.

Pins and Needles

Almost everyone has had a hand or foot 'go to sleep'. Usually this sensation is due to pressure on a limb's blood vessels and nerves and represents your body's way of crying 'Give in!' The pins-and-needles feeling passes after the pressure is relieved by uncrossing your legs, or by your brand new lover waking up and getting off your arm.

But what if your hand went to sleep and never woke up? Next time, before the sensation passes, remember that this sort of numbness can be an early sign of leprosy.

Most people think they have come no closer to leprosy than watching reruns of Ben Hur. Few realize that there are still ten to twenty million lepers in the world. The chief areas of concentration in the U.K. are those occupied by people who are rich enough, and foolish enough, to take extended holidays in 'exotic' locations.

The first signs are usually patches that are darker or lighter than the surrounding skin, but many cases begin with areas of numbness. These changes are due to infiltration of the skin by the bacteria, *Mycobacteria leprae* – a distant cousin of the organisms that cause tuberculosis, though neither will own up to the relationship. Fingers and nose fall off sometime thereafter.

Cases of advanced leprosy are rarely seen today and this disease is now less a medical than a psychological danger. Effective drug therapy is widely available, and researchers have found that leprosy can be communicated to another only after prolonged exposure. Etiquette books continue to suggest that if your date complains that her foot has fallen asleep, you should wave goodbye through tinted glass instead of kissing her goodnight; today such recommendations may be overly cautious.

Nevertheless, the social stigma surrounding this disease persists, and a sudden cry of 'Leper!' will still empty a cinema. Leprosy's victims are understandably touchy on this issue. They have organized themselves into support groups that offer psychological counselling and are now campaigning to change the name of their affliction from leprosy to the less familiar and less inflammatory 'Hansen's Disease.' Don't be fooled.

Frequent Urination

This problem comes up all the time and is suffered by people of all ages: the child who makes his father stop the car half-a-dozen times on the M5; the student taking an exam who makes four trips to the lavatory thereby provoking charges that he is cheating; the young woman who excuses herself over and over during the course of the evening, leaving her date to wonder – 'Can this be normal?'

Incredibly, the answer is yes.

How often someone needs to do what doctors call 'number one' depends on many factors, including the volume of fluid the person drinks and how much of it includes caffeine, since that increases urine output. Coffee has cut short thousands of conversations, while Cola spoiled *Gone With the Wind* for a generation of film fans. And, of course, we all know the effect of alcohol on urination, which is well-summarized in the

First Law of Kidney Physiology – 'You don't buy beer; you rent it.'

Like so many bodily functions, increased frequency of urination can be an early warning sign of a serious illness or – more likely – evidence that it is already too late. Thus, careful patients should keep track of the time, amount, and general quality of each voiding and insist on discussing this data with their doctors once a week.

While no one really knows how many trips to the loo per day are 'normal' – a value-laden term and a concept that has outlived its usefulness – most doctors accept the following:

1.   The adult male bladder holds about one pint of urine and the female bladder slightly less. Some patients do have a diminished capacity, but not all of them have cancer.

2.   The average urine output per twenty-four hours is about three pints.

3.   For comfort, for dignity, and sometimes just for something to do, most adults void when their bladder is half-full (or half-empty, if you wish); this adds up to five or six times each day.

4.   If we assume about one minute for every voiding, then the average person spends three months of his life urinating and six months washing his hands afterwards.

In other words, we 'piss away' as it were, a period equivalent to our last year at college – for many of us the best year of our lives. Those who void more often are losing even more precious time – yet another reason to carefully monitor this important bodily function.

The most common cause of excessive urination in women is an infection of the urinary tract, a well-known variant of which is 'honeymoon cystitis.' The infection begins in these women shortly after sexual intercourse; it seems that during all the

21

commotion down there, bacteria climb up into the bladder. Decades of research and millions of pounds have been spent in study of this problem , but our understanding of it has progressed little beyond the conclusions of the anatomists who originally described the syndrome – 'God put the waterworks too close to the playground.'

Unfortunately, increase frequency of urination can also herald the onset of more serious diseases. Some of them are common, such as diabetes mellitus. In patients afflicted with this complaint, a high blood sugar level robs the kidney of the ability to concentrate urine. Thus, the diabetic finds himself constantly urinating and constantly drinking to make up for water lost. The sugar that is 'spilled' during output makes the urine sweet to the taste – the oldest way of diagnosing diabetes. (This technique has been replaced by modern technology, thank God.)

A rare form of diabetes, diabetes insipidus, has nothing to do with high blood sugar. This illness is caused by tumours of the pituitary gland, which is located in a rather sensitive area of the brain about two inches behind the eyes. As these tumours grow, they destroy cells that produce a hormone needed by your kidneys to concentrate urine. Without the hormone, you urinate five gallons a day or more of almost pure water. In the Middle East these patients are admired for their ability to make the desert bloom, but elsewhere this condition has its drawbacks.

These tumours also press on other structures, especially the optic nerves. Usually, the first deficit that evolves is loss of peripheral vision. So if you are urinating more and enjoying it less, ask yourself:

1. Do I get headaches?
2. Am I having trouble seeing things way off to the side?

If the answer to both these questions is no, then the chances that you have a pituitary tumour are slightly reduced.

The Sniffles

A runny nose, or rhinitis, is usually due to a cold or exposure to an allergen, such as pollen. Its consequence is generally limited to making you an unpopular person to sit with for more than thirty seconds.

Sometimes, though, rhinitis is prolonged and can signal a sinus infection or more serious condition. Among these are Lethal Midline Granuloma (described in slightly more detail under *Ten Diseases You Were Better Off Not Knowing About*); Wegener's Granulomatosis (an inflammatory disease that can erode the nasal septum and damage the lungs and kidneys); congenital syphilis; and leprosy. None of these is going to help you win friends and influence people.

Then there is the possibility that what is running out of your nose and onto your sleeve is not mucus at all, but cerebrospinal fluid – the clear liquid that surrounds and bathes the brain. If the skull is fractured, cerebrospinal fluid can leak out into the nose. The danger lies not in loss of the fluid, but in the spread of bacteria from the nose into the brain. What then ensues is the micro-organisms's equivalent of the Oktoberfest.

Doctors have a quick test to distinguish cerebrospinal fluid from mucus – they just measure the liquid's protein levels, which will be quite high if the liquid is mucus. So if you are concerned by your runny nose, simply mail a sample of your discharge to your doctor. He will be glad to tell you whether he thinks you should have your head examined.

Night Blindness

Patients constantly wonder whether they are getting enough vitamins. They are especially concerned about vitamin A, because 'A' comes at the beginning of the alphabet, suggesting that this vitamin must have unusual importance.

And they are right. Vitamin A, which is found in many vegetables, is crucial to normal vision. True deficiencies usually manifest themselves first with a complaint of night blindness, and can almost always be traced to dietary inadequacies or gastrointestinal diseases causing an inability to absorb the vitamin. Irreversible damage to vision will occur if these problems are not corrected.

So when patients say they are concerned about their vitamin A level, we suggest that they ask themselves, 'Do I have trouble seeing in the dark?' If the answer is yes, they may be vitamin A deficient and should consider supplementation, or at least eating some vegetables once in a while. Just don't overdo it. Vitamin A overdoses can be dangerous, and patients taking it should be on the alert for the signs of toxicity—headaches, loss of hair, kidney and liver damage and birth defects.

After offering this advice, we tell patients that they are on their own.

Excess Saliva

Production of too much saliva, also known as 'ptyalism', is often ascribed by laymen of carelessness or lack of control. In fact, ptyalism can be a manifestation of a number of illnesses that affect salivation nerve centres located in the lower brainstem. Drooling can be induced by encephalitis (inflammation of the brain), rabies, botulism, arsenic poisoning, or rare degenerative nerve diseases. Any of these possesses the ability to transform one's mind into something resembling anchovy paste.

If you are not sure whether you suffer from ptyalism, spit one day's production of saliva into a container and send it to your doctor. If you use a messenger service, you can be sure it will get there overnight. Repeat once a week as a precaution until your doctor promises you will never become ill, or until he is forced to move to an area not covered by messenger services. If you do turn out to have ptyalism, there is only one way to spell relief: L-o-u-r-d-e-s.

Ringing in the Ears

Tinnitus, or ringing in the ears, is usually due to wax in the ear's external canal. That is a disgusting enough situation for anyone to confront, not to mention embarrassing for everyone involved. Most doctors are more at ease telling a patient he has cancer than an earful of wax.

Still, doctors wish that all cases of tinnitus were due to ear wax – life would be so much simpler. If a patient came in complaining of ringing in the ears, we'd know that we should not examine them without rubber gloves. Unfortunately, almost any disorder of the ear can cause this problem, including infections and trauma from noise at work and rock concerts.

The most feared cause of tinnitus is a tumour of the nerve to the ear – an acoustic neuroma. Because of the strategic location of this nerve inside the skull, these tumours can raise a lot of hell if allowed to grow. Fully excluding this possibility requires a rather expensive set of X-rays involving considerable radiation exposure and personal attention.

Go for it.

Headaches

Rare as brain tumours are, almost everyone has heard a horror story like that concerning George Gershwin. One day, the great composure of 'Rhapsody in Blue' had a headache; the next, some difficulty in finishing a concert. A few months later, he was dead from a glioblastoma. People like George Gershwin give headaches a bad name.

Actually, most headaches don't have anything to do with the brain, other than being at the same end of the body. They arise from tension of the muscles under the scalp and face or, as in migraine headaches, spasms of blood vessels in the head. Bad as they are, they eventually pass.

There are, however, a number of serious and potentially fatal causes which the layman couldn't possibly separate from the common or garden variety induced by screeching children. Among them are brain tumours, meningitis, and end-stage syphilis.

Bad as these disorders are, doctors are troubled even more by the fear that a headache may represent a subdural hematoma. These hematomas, or blood clots, begin with a tear of the veins inside the skull, usually after head trauma. This trauma can be as mild as bumping one's head on the bottom of the dinner table while picking up a dropped fork. The torn veins will usually repair themselves, but sometimes they continue to leak and the clot slowly expands. Eventually, the brain gets squeezed over to one side, or out of the hole in the bottom. Not surprisingly, this pressure causes headaches.

In one case, a nearly fatal subdural was attributed to a fall on the ice almost twenty-five years before the clot was finally detected. Of course, if you haven't bumped your head in the last quarter century you have little to worry about. As a precaution, we personally never pick up eating implements we drop at dinner. We don't get invited back often, but we sleep better at night for it.

Head Size

Is your head too large?

If so, you may have Paget's Disease, a bone disorder

found in about three percent of patients over the age of forty. In this poorly-understood disease, normal bone is replaced by abnormal, poorly-formed and bulkier bone – sometimes in one or two areas, occasionally everywhere.

Most patients never know they have Paget's Disease, but others notice a swelling or deformity of a limb and may limp as one leg lengthens. Those with Paget's of the skull find that their hat size increases. Later, severe headaches occur and the new bone can choke off nerves from the brain to the ear. Occasionally, bone at the base of the skull compresses the spinal cord, leading to paralysis.

Promising treatments for Paget's disease are now under development, making it worthwhile for you to check your own skull circumference periodically. Weekly measurements plotted on a graph can be very helpful to your doctor.

Hiccups

Hiccups represent a complex reflex that follows irritation of the respiratory muscles – especially the diaphragm – or the nerves connecting them with the brain. Most episodes have no obvious cause and pass after several uncomfortable and embarrassing hours during which your closest friends will avoid you.

Occasionally, though, hiccups are a sign that something more ominous is afoot, in which case we call them 'hiccoughs.' Pneumonia and liver tumours can both irritate the diaphragm, while brain tumours and viral enciphalitis – infections of the brain – can induce hiccoughs from above. Heart attacks involving the bottom of the heart, which rests on the diaphragm, can also produce hiccoughs. Sometimes, these humiliating little noises are the first sign of heart disease.

Some people like to try curing hiccups by scaring the

patient with sudden noises. These tactics usually work in some cases. You should keep in mind, however, that if the patient is indeed having a heart attack you might just kill him.

Drowsiness

If you have become drowsy while reading this section, do not be alarmed. Sleepiness is experienced by most people much of the time, and by certain politicians almost all the time. It is particularly associated with the alpha and omega of human existence – sexual intercourse and large meals – both of which should immediately be followed by a long nap. The unifying theme in these superficially disparate activities is that of movement: movement of the earth during the former, movement of the colon during the latter. (In an unfortunate few, movement of the earth during climax and of the colon during digestion are functionally linked. These were the ones who were asked to leave Boy Scout Camp within a week of their arrival).

Drowsiness during other activities, such as watching the Eurovision Song Contest or listening to Today in Parliament, may be a warning that you are about to die in your sleep. This fate is particularly frightening, because it cruelly denies the patient one of life's most fulfilling moments: telling the doctor he was wrong when he said you didn't have a fatal disease.

For example, you could be coming down with St. Louis encephalitis, an infection by a virus that feeds on your frontal lobes. Contrary to popular belief, you can't get it from a toilet seat. The virus is carried by mosquitoes, who leave it behind when they bite. Then the microbes travel right to your head, and proceed to disassemble your silicon chips. By the time they finish, your brain looks like a neurological version of Liverpool 8. The expression 'Room at the Top' takes on new meanings for you and your friends.

More popular causes of drowsiness are failures of the liver (cirrhosis) and of the kidney. When those organs precede you across the Great Divide, the poisons they normally clear from your blood are sopped up by your brain like dirty dishwater in a paper towel. It is an ironic commentary on our state of evolution that anything we can't urinate immediately gets stored in the brain. This phenomenon may be the best explanation for the condition of the present Government.

Then there's the Kleine-Levin Syndrome. This extremely rare disorder has no known cause and tends to attack younger people. It is manifested by recurrent episodes of sleepiness, excessive hunger, restlessness, irritability, and a destructive degree of mental confusion. It is sometimes mistaken for a much more common – and more painful – malady: male adolescence. There is no cure for victims of either disorder. They should be put to sleep by a veterinary surgeon amid peaceful surroundings.

Blue Navel

The navel is an often unappreciated feature of the otherwise bland expanse of one's abdomen. Like those Swiss weather prediction toys (when the gnome is pink, it's going to rain; when the gnome is black, sell gold) it can be a beacon that signals the inner chaos of your intestines.

A suddenly blue navel, for instance, is typically regarded by patients as a laughable curiosity: something to show the boss during a dull lunch hour. In reality, a blue navel can signify either of two impending disasters. It can mean that there is a large amount of blood in your abdomen due to the rupture of a big, big blood vessel. In this case, forget about impressing the boss; you're not going to collect your bonus.

Alternatively, a blue navel can mean you have

pancreatitis, an inflammation of the gland behind your stomach that looks like polystyrene chips but is actually vital to normal digestion. Usually, pancreatitis is due to over-indulgence in alcohol. A pancreas exposed to too much alcohol can blow up faster than a cockroach in a microwave oven.[1]

Our advice to patients is this: after a two-bottle lunch with an important client or the company chairman, take off your shirt, or unzip your dress, and quickly check the colour of your navel. A little forethought on your part will allow you to plan the rest of the day or evening around a possible trip to an emergency department. If you are drinking during an evening of romance, a navel check may well start the ball rolling, especially if it is presented in the context of preventive medicine.

Fatigue

Fatigue is a normal physiological response to exertion, mental or physical. But it is also a normal physiological response to poisoning with *Clostridium botulinum* – better known as botulism.

As everyone who gets a little nervous about vichyssoise or corned beef knows, botulism is transmitted in improperly canned foods. The clostridia bacteria secrete a powerful toxin that usually dissolves in prolonged, intense heat. Sometimes, though, a breakdown in the heating process allows the poison to survive. The results are deadly.

Fatigue develops first, usually about one day after exposure. Eventually, neuromuscular disturbances lead to double vision, difficulty in swallowing or talking, and weakness. Typically, the mind remains clear to the end. Two-thirds of cases are fatal.

In the U.K., the most common sources of botulism

---

1. Thirteen seconds.

are tinned vegetables, seafood, pork and beef. Because of this, doctors are given to telling patients to avoid these foods in any form, tinned or fresh. Instead they should choose their foods from one of these five basic groups.

1. Encapsulated foods. Health food shops offer a variety of tasty snacks and gourmet dinners in handy tablet or capsule form.

2. Foods like coleslaw or organic egg salad that have no shape or definable colour or taste. Available at the same shops.

3. Food that cannot be easily separated from its wrapper. If you have trouble getting through, it is going to be much harder for germs which have no hands and a poor sense of direction.

4. Foods derived from petroleum byproducts rather than grown in dirty dirt. Once available only along major motorways, such foods are now to be found all over the country.

5. Chilli.

If you insist on purchasing a tinned product, take a bradawl to the supermarket. Stick it into your prospective purchase and hold the can up to your ear to listen for escaping gas. Hold a match near the hole. Shake the can and look for foam. Do not buy any can that emits flammable gas when punctured. If the supermarket employees approach you with a few questions, wave the bradawl wildly at them.

Irritability

Though irritability among many of our readers is perfectly understandable, it is sometimes more justified than they might guess. Serious brain disorders or accumulations of toxins can produce alterations in mood or personality-changes, many of which may initially seem improvements. Patients will often think that they are just out-of-sorts, or have turned over a new leaf, when in fact they will soon be pushing up daisies. Such cases give rise to the medical dictum, 'A new you may be the last you.'

Specifically, irritability could be an early sign of rabies or tetanus – two diseases that would have been invented by parents to terrify children had they not already existed. Grouchy patients should regularly search their homes and workplaces for rusty objects upon which they might have cut themselves. They should also examine their dogs daily for evidence of excessive drooling.

Sweating

There is little good to say about sweat. Even in a normal, healthy person, perspiration is dangerous. Apart from the devastation it wreaks on social intercourse, there is the constant threat of dehydration and electrolyte disturbances that cause fainting spells and even cardiac arrests. Fear of these consequences explains why most doctors avoid any activity likely to produce perspiration.

If the picture painted by the information in this chapter has depressed you, well, it should. If history has taught us anything, it's that everything can be bad news. Even feeling good can be bad. Patients occasionally glide into our offices exuding a sense of well-being, of fulfillment, of confidence in their physical and mental health. All too often, this euphoria is the beginning of the end.

Many deadly diseases are capable of producing a giddiness that patients confuse with that much rarer entity, true happiness. They might, for example, be harbouring adrenal or pituitary tumours that secrete toxic levels of corticosteroids, causing a 'steroid high' that fills the patient with a mysterious energy and ironic joy.

32

Inappropriate elation can also mean that the brain is running on too little oxygen — suggesting major problems with the heart and lungs. High concentrations of oxygen may bring these patients back to earth, but the underlying diseases are usually so serious that resuming a normal life is out of the question. Patients remain on the ground only for a brief refuelling before continuing their flights. So if you find yourself feeling extraordinarily well, we recommend getting to a hospital immediately. It may already be too late.

3
Life threatening infections you can catch from your pets

I had a dog, his name was Blue,
Bet you five dollars he was a good dog, too.
— Deservedly Anon. Folk Song

Right. And *we'll* bet you twice the amount that Blue, if given the opportunity, would have turned his master in to the police for a plane ticket to the Carribean and the companionship of a saucy French poodle.

We've made a lot of money this way, because most people live in a fantasy world when it comes to their pets. They ignore the dark side to our dealings with pets — the reasons we sometimes call them 'animals'.

We don't want to overstate the danger, or imply that we think pets are intrinsically evil. After all, they're not so clever; in the final analysis, a dog is a dog, and a horse is a horse. But doctors also know that every interaction between Man And The Beast That Does Tricks Sometimes, is like playing in traffic. Animals harbour a variety of parasites that can turn your organs into diet cola, rob you of your intellect, and put the rest of you in a medical doggy bag. No wonder, then, that most of our patients have been wary of their pets since childhood and they usually trace the fears to seeing the Disney classic *Old Yeller* – a traumatic childhood experience rivalled only by birth, puberty, and the divorce of one's parents.

In case you've repressed the memory, Old Yeller was a dog who gave pieces of his tattered yellow hide in reckless endeavours like fighting grizzly bears. His courage was exceeded only by his ability to absorb punishment. Indeed, he has been the inspiration for countless white boxers.

These tactics quickly removed our hero from the ranks of All Things Bright and Beautiful, and turned from him Young Yeller to Old Yeller by the age of two, which is like being fourteen years old for a human being according to the theory of relativity. Not pretty and not very bright, Yeller's fierce loyalty nevertheless won him a place in a pioneer family, not to mention our hearts. (Yeller was a bit of a pioneer himself. He was the first 'ugly' dog to make it big anywhere but the living room rug, shattering the show dog mould of Lassie and Rin Tin Tin. In his day, he was the Barbra Streisand of the Disney kennels.)

The rest is history. A rabid wolf attacked the family. Old Yeller fought it off, absorbing his usual beating and contracting rabies to boot. Since veterinary surgeons had not yet invented the after-dinner speech, the family's son had to put him to sleep by shooting him with something resembling a bazooka – several times as we recall, though perhaps it was only the report of a single shot that has echoed in our memories for years.

As boy and dog stared at each other along the barrel of the gun, all parties had a better understanding of the word 'ambivalence.' The boy was learning that sometimes you have to give up the things you love most, and occasionally that means shooting them. Old Yeller, who had quickly considered all avenues of escape and saw that it was hopeless, realised that he should have bitten the hand that fed him while he could. As for us – the eleven year-olds in the audience who would always consider Old Yeller far more deserving of our tears than Ali Magraw at her best – we were awash with emotion. We were wondering what kind of man Walt Disney was to let this happen. We were asking our parents why doctors couldn't cure rabies with a pill or something. And, above all, we were thinking about that big dog down the street that had been drooling on our sandals and wondering what would happen to us if *we* got rabies.

Thus we learned that pets bring many things into our lives, and that some of them are fatal diseases. Despite *Old Yeller*, dogs account for many of the more than one hundred and fifty diseases that can be transmitted to humans.

Of course, lots of these diseases are minor skin infections, like Puppy Dog Dermatitis. This infestation by *Sarcoptes scabiei* produces an intensely itchy scaling rash that your doctor will poke at with a Q-tip while breathing through his mouth before packing you off to the dermatologist. These illnesses usually respond to treatments that fall far short of actually shooting the dog.

The other infections carried by dogs, cats, fish and birds can transform your body into the ecological equivalent of Bonio.

A selection follows.

Salmonellosis

In 1975, the American Food and Drug Administration banned interstate trafficking in pet turtles. What did this mean? True, the FBI had fallen on hard times – embarrassed by Watergate and overwhelmed by the narcotics industry, it needed some easier assignments to recoup its reputation. But still, your average pet shop owner is a far cry from Dillinger, and photographs of G–men posing beside confiscated turtles failed to fire anyone's imagination. No wonder the TV series was cancelled.

There was actually a good reason for the ban. More than half of pet turtles are carriers of the bacteria *Salmonella* which causes millions of cases of gastroenteritis each year – more, in fact, than the entire export total of Benidorm and Marbella combined. Many patients have fifty or more bowel movements per day, far exceeding nursery guidelines. Very young or old patients often become so dehydrated they pass out; some cases are even fatal. Countless others merely wish they were dead, but are forced to endure two weeks of misery before recovering.

The American ban on pet turtles caused a seventy-seven percent decline in salmonella infections from turtle-associated strains of the bug, but the disease remains common because so many other animals carry the bacteria. About twelve percent of cats are infected, as well as twenty percent of dogs. Salmonella is also common among the chicks and ducklings that many children find so attractive. These cuddly balls of fluff realize that they have only a few weeks to live and the bacteria represents their best hope of taking a child or two with them.

Bubonic Plague

Examining what the cat dragged in has long been a ritual in everyday life. Many potential doctors lost interest in anatomy while poking a stick at the remains of a field mouse left on the doormat.[1] Disgust, though, was usually tempered by admiration for an animal that

---

1. Many families mistakenly interpret this gesture as a form of tribute. Actually, anthropologists believe that it is just convenient, and is the evolutionary forerunner of leaving your books on the kitchen table when you come home from school, or throwing your clothes on the only chair in the bedroom.

slept on windowsills most of the day, lived off the land at night, and could get away with almost anything on the grounds that it is in heat.

We would have felt a little differently had we realized that the cat might be bringing home bubonic plague, better known as 'The Black Death.'

Which Black Death, you ask? The same Black Death that swept the world in the 6th century, the 14th century, and, to a lesser extent, at the end of the 19th century; that has frightened and inspired authors from Dionysius to Camus; that most doctors refer to as *the* plague. *That* Black Death is alive and well and could be living almost anywhere. In fact, bubonic plague never really disappeared. Cases have appeared sporadically for years, though most have been too mild to be reported.

Today, doctors understand that the disease is caused not by religious indiscretion, but by a bacteria called *Yersinia pestis*. This bug is carried by fleas and frequently attacks small animals, especially rats, squirrels and rabbits.

Contact with these animals leads to infection in an occasional boy scout or nature-lover. They make their beds; they can lie in them. But, at the edge of town, these fleas also attack 'city-mice' and pets, eventually bringing the Black Death to normal people minding their own business. Although antibiotics can curb cases if used early enough, and vaccines make another major epidemic unlikely, sporadic cases will almost surely continue to pop up, so a few common-sense precautions seem in order:

1.   Never pet a rat without boiling it first.
2.   Never kiss a squirrel on the lips.
3.   Wear a flea collar around the house or to any setting where you are likely to encounter other living things.
4.   Always remember that a rabbit is not a toy. It is a shy, graceful creature that would like to see you swell up and die.

Cat Scratch Disease

Cat Scratch Disease is a prototype for pet-related illnesses in two key ways:

1. You feel terrible once the illness has set in.
2. The animal feels perfectly fine.

In fact, the cat is not ill at all. It is only carrying a virus on its paws. This virus will not infect the cat, but *will* slip inside you when kitty takes a playful slash at your face as you try to put the catnip away. A week or so later, lymph nodes in your armpits, neck, and groin swell up and start to drain pus, at which point your lover may become a bit suspicious about where those scratches really came from.

The lumps themselves are not hazardous. If left alone, the swollen nodes and the washed-out feeling that accompanies them leave with hardly a trace, much like your ex-lover. The main danger is that they will be mistaken for lymphomas or other tumours requiring surgery. Many patients have had 'cancers' removed by a surgeon, only to find that their lumps were just another form of kitty litter. While recovering from surgery, patients often ask what kind of ballast cats make and whether a Dobermann can be taught to climb trees.

Although we deplore this sudden hostility toward cats, we are not really surprised by it. After all, people who own cats are usually a little weird. Deprived of ordinary human friendship, they put all their emotional eggs into the single basket of their relationships with their cats. And yet they are the first to reach for a strychnine-filled mouse when the cat opens up an artery, or curls up on their faces as they sleep.

It's not the cat's fault – his brain is just the size of a walnut, so how much mischief can he deliberately make? He just wants attention. A little patience and a few simple rules will allow you and your cat to grow old together, free of parasites and unwanted visits from relatives and friends.

Don't let your pet have too much responsibility too early. Pushing it to grow up will only make it unhappy. Exert some control over your cat's television habits. Be especially sure the set is off when you are both eating your dinners, even if you use separate cans. Don't overburden your cat with your adult problems. All too often, people use their pets as therapists or confidantes, forgetting a single important fact — a cat is really stupid. He doesn't understand what you are saying. He doesn't want to hear about your neuroses; he wants to claw up the couch.

If none of these suggestions work, and your cat continues to show signs of hostility, we suggest:

1. Getting out the lead booties and enrolling him in swimming classes.
2. Or taking him out for 'dinner' at a Chinese restaurant. It will be the meal of his life.

Babesiosis

Suddenly, being chic is chic again. Rich people are feeling good about themselves. They aren't ashamed of having a lot of money, or time spent at prep school, or owning people. They're proud of their portfolios and, if they have babesiosis, they tell the world about it.

Babesiosis, you see, is the disease of the elite — and why not? Other classes have *their* own diseases — sickle cell anemia, for example. In contrast, babesiosis isn't even something you can inherit. Most cases have been caught in one very special place — the exclusive resort of Nantucket. Thus, to have this disease is to signal the world that you spend the summer there and that, sick as you are, you still have more money, influence and good taste than they ever will.

One clear advantage in having babesiosis is that you look as pale and drawn as a *Vogue* model. Other aspects aren't as advantageous. Blood counts fall, while your body is wracked by fever, chills, muscle aches and nausea. The sense of fullness in your belly means that your spleen has swollen to deal with the infection. Patients often complain of a sense of *weltschmerz* in the late stages, though we suspect that it is usually affected.

Ironically, the earliest recorded victims of this infection were beasts of burden – Verse 3, Chapter 9 of Exodus describes a divine plague of cattle and pets in Egypt that probably represented babesiosis.

The illness is caused by a small parasite that invades red blood cells, a parasite which is carried from animal to animal by ticks. Sometimes, those ticks mistake rich people for their pets. The resulting illness can take you from the social register to a *Times* obituary within a matter of weeks.

So when you return from holiday and your suntan is beginning to fade, keep the glow alive by telling your friends that you feel tired and have been running a temperature. Mention the drenching sweats and your aching muscles. Throw up on the floor. Finally, drop the news that your spleen is enlarging. They'll die of jealousy.

By the way, there's no treatment.

Toxoplasmosis

Toxoplasma gondii is not an obscure Indian pacifist; it is a parasite that lives in about half of us and is yet another reason to distrust cats. This bug is carried around by domestic felines as well as cougars, wild cats, and Asian leopards. Cats excrete the parasite's eggs everywhere: into the soil, the water, the living room rug. From there, they are picked up by all kinds of animals, including rugby players. Thus about ten percent of the lamb and a quarter of the pork sold in this country contain the eggs. If these meats are eaten while undercooked, toxoplasmosis follows.

Inside the body, the egg hatches and grows into a form called the trophozoite – much as depicted in the movie *Alien*. The trophozoite is as cute as a button, and will go anywhere in the body to play. It's favourite haunts are the lymph glands, which swell into hard lumps. Most infections are mild, with only one or two lumps and associated symptoms like fatigue, malaise, headache and mild abdominal pains – about what one experiences during an income tax audit.

Occasionally, the germ spreads everywhere and your body gets so lumpy that it resembles a rosary. That's just what you may need when the germ invades the heart, lungs, and particularly the membrane that covers the brain, which may eventually have to be shipped to Lourdes under separate cover.

There are a few simple precautions that you can take to ensure safety from *Toxoplasma gondii*:

1. Get rid of your Asian leopard immediately. Just untie it and let it go. It will soon become someone else's problem.
2. Cook all meat, particularly cat meat, until it is black in the middle. Serve plain, or on a bed of wild rice.
3. Thoroughly wash and then bury all garden-grown vegetables without eating them.
4. Clean kitty litter boxes with napalm or some other government approved bleach.

The picture we have painted is a grim one. And we have not even mentioned psittacosis, a pneumonia caught from birds (and the most difficult disease to pronounce without spitting). Tulmaremia, a systemic illness carried by rabbits; or the self-explanatory toxacara viscera larva migrans. Still, we feel that the capacity of your pet to transform you from a taxpayer into a deduction on someone else's tax return does not demand a tough attitude toward all animals.

No doubt some animals deserve it. Roy Rogers stuffed and mounted Bullet and Trigger for offences that could only be hinted at. But recent statistics suggest that our relationships with pets may be less dangerous than associations with other human beings.

Dog bites were down 16.7% in 1980 in comparison with the previous year, for example. The number of incidents of humans biting other humans increased by twenty-four percent over the same period. In fact, bites from every species except humans declined.

Examination of the data reveals even more depressing trends. Individuals in the twenty-twenty-five year-old group received the most human bites; right behind them were the fifteen – twenty year-olds. That college age and secondary school age individuals should lead the pack in getting bitten says something sad about the quality of education in this country. No wonder little Johnny can't read; he can't even keep his hand out of someone else's mouth.

Even more dispiriting is the statistic that tells us that while half of the bites were classified as 'aggressive,' almost forty percent of the bites were attributed to 'unknown' activities. It seems that these people cannot recall how they came to be chewed!

Most disturbing in this mournful litany is the fact that five percent of all human bites were caused by children biting their doctors. We recommend that such children receive a radical medical therapy administered by trained specialists. It's technical name is 'The Old Yeller Treatment.'

4
Physical fitness is hazardous to your health

I'm not feeling so good.
    — Alberto Salazar, after winning the 1982 Boston Marathon

Western culture thrives on the marriage of ideas. Still, we are more than a little puzzled by the current confusion of perspiration with recreation. We understand the joys of competition. Even for us, the thrill of victory has its allure. But the agony of the feet — and virtually everything else — is another matter, usually medical. We've taken care of too many javelin wounds to ignore the obvious: physical fitness is hazardous to your health. Few things in life are as dangerous as good clean fun.

We were especially concerned a year or so ago when two leading newspapers ran major articles on the fitness boom, transforming it from a mere trend into a bonafide fad. It recalled for us the horror of the early sixties. That turbulent decade witnessed the birth of fifty-mile walks, folk dancing, and the first outbreak of jogging, which spread rapidly despite intensive aerial spraying of runners. There was an upsurge in active sports like swimming, touch football, and running for

Parliament, accompanied by the decline of more cerebral pastimes like Monopoly, pinball, and locking your sister in the cupboard. Abdomens were flat. Spirits were flatter. It had to stop.

Just in time, God provided *Superstars*. Some of you may be unfamiliar with this institution because you have been living in a cave in Tibet. The rest of us know that this show provides the opportunity to watch athletes with muscles in their earlobes performing acts of strength and skill so demanding that even the viewer can barely summon the energy to lift his can of *Long Life*. More pleasing to the armchair spectator is the fact that the participants are often required to compete in events other than those in which they excel, thereby allowing the viewer to sneer at the patent amateurishness of some jock attempting to acquit himself decently in a kyak event despite the fact that he's an aquaphobic non-swimmer whose only talent is for the hammer-throw.

The attractiveness of the show lies, partially, in the packaging. Even more important, though, was the TV company's insight that men everywhere had grown tired of winning, losing, or making any kind of effort. They wanted a graceful way out: an excuse to stay indoors, downing beers, and pretending that with a week or so's training they could compete in *Superstars* themselves.

In general, doctors were delighted with this trend toward armchair (as opposed to wheelchair) participation. True, business fell off for orthopaedic surgeons and psychiatrists began to diagnose strange new psychoses.[1] In addition, irreparable damage was done

---

1. Unhealthy preoccupations with parrots and vomit were sometimes reported, together with a tendency in some male patients to remove their partial dentures and have their hair permed. A study undertaken in 1980 showed that some viewers exhibited homicidal behaviour-patterns during televised athletics meetings. This was later formally termed 'Coleman syndrome.'

to the English language by people called 'commentators'. All things considered, though, people seemed safer sitting in front of their television set than running around a field like demented goats.[1]

Unfortunately, though, watching sports may be an activity whose time has come and gone. Physical fitness itself is back with a vengeance – and the evidence can be found in casualty departments everywhere. People are once again taking to the open air, killing themselves in an attempt to live longer. When they go shopping, they are apt to buy Japanese running shoes instead of British beer, thus worsening the national trade deficit.

Doctors regard all this activity with a bloodshot eye. Most medical men simply don't like sports. We are still bitter about being stuck in goal during school soccer matches which, at that level of play, is like being appointed ambassador to Nepal – little responsibility but less fun, and no one notices you until you make a mess of things. Besides, professional restrictions and the Road Traffic Act require doctors to use golf carts in those rare situations where a Mercedes is inappropriate – like going out to close the garden-gate.

We'll admit that there are some benefits to the running boom – for example, more young women are wearing sleeveless T-shirts and thin cotton shorts in public than ever before. But, as doctors, we can see people without *any* clothes on *whenever we want*! So most of us have stuck by our old hobbies, like building tax shelters in bottles. Doctors who do indulge in sports choose those where the odds dictate that they will not be the ones who get hurt – hunting, for example. All other athletic activity is considered dangerous.

Thus we feel a responsibility to let the public know

---

1.   These conclusions were drawn before doctors understood the radiation involved in watching television. See Chapter 4 in *The Hypochondriac's Handbook*, Vol II.

just how dangerous fitness can be. You don't need a government health warning to tell you about the obvious hazards involved in some sports. Everyone knows about 'Sky Diver's Earache' and the nosebleeds that plague mountain climbers. But you ought to be aware of the subtle, rare, and all too real complications of modern life in general, and sports in particular, that have recently appeared in the medical literature. The columns of medical journals are overflowing with horror stories about activities that once seemed safe . . .

The Case Against Running

The earliest case report demonstrating the hazards of running comes down to us from the Persian Wars. In 490 B.C., in the wake of the Athenian victory over the army of Datis at Marathon, a Greek runner named Pheidippides was dispatched with news of the triumph. He reached Athens, but never got to the post-script. Still, in his final act he did communicate an even more important message – running can make you drop dead.

Since then, a variety of subtler complications have been described by doctors in an attempt to dissuade their patients from running themselves into the ground, so to speak. For example, we have cautioned our patients that the common practice among marathoners of dabbing benzene-containing rubber cement on their feet to cushion blisters can cause anemia, or even leukemia. They were undeterred until we pointed out that having leukemia could adversely affect their times. Virtually all our other warnings have been ignored, strengthening our suspicion that the runner's brain suffers thousands of tiny concussions as he bounces along. Were this not the case, then many would have given up the 'sport' after hearing of 'Penile

Frostbite: An Unforeseen Hazard of Jogging,' as reported recently in one of our foremost journals of medicine.

The case concerned a doctor who went out for a routine thirty minute run in mid-December. The temperature was 18°F; a biting east wind made it seem even colder. Five minutes before the end of the run, the doctor noted 'an unpleasant painful burning sensation at the penile tip . . . the pain increasing with each stride.'

On examining himself at home, the doctor was horrified to discover early frostbite of the penis. Fortunately, rapid therapy produced a complete cure. It would be in bad taste to provide details of either treatment or response, though a videotape is available to special customers.

Almost as frightening is 'Jogger's Nipple' – a painful breast abrasion produced by repeated rubbing against a shirt – usually the runner's own. Originally, this syndrome was distressingly common among serious women runners. For example fifteen percent of the female runners in the first Chicago Marathon reported 'chafing.'

Since then, most women runners have learned to prevent such problems with petroleum jelly or protective shields we doctors call 'pasties'. Thus, most current victims of this syndrome are male.

Men and women alike are subject to the indignities of the gastrointestinal complications of running, as reviewed by Dr. Stephen N. Sullivan of Victoria Hospital in Ontario, Canada. He surveyed fifty-seven long distance runners and found plenty of evidence that the legs aren't the only part of the anatomy in movement. Among his findings:

— Ten percent reported heartburn when running.
— Thirty percent occasionally or frequently had the urge or need to defecate, often forcing what is called 'a nip into the bushes.'

— A quarter had cramps or diarrhoea after competitive running. 'Only six percent had severe nausea or retching,' he added.

Only?

Our response, as members of a profession devoted even more to avoiding pain than relieving it, is to ask why, if God had meant us to run, did he give us the Porsche?

Waterskier's Enema

On the surface, waterskiing seems a perfect sport for the medical profession. To begin with, you have to be rich to play it. Just as important, it doesn't demand much teamwork. In fact, it doesn't take much more than staying on your feet, hanging on, and pretending you're not bored by going around in circles. These tasks should pose no problems for anyone in private practice.

But, as with most endeavours in which taking off one's glasses is recommended, there are hidden dangers. Drowning, for one. Shark attack for another. In some European waterways, where speedboats criss-cross like dragonfly, there is also the constant threat of U-boat Syndrome, in which the victim is run down by a German submarine.

You can add to these the risk of waterskier's enema and waterskier's douche, most often suffered by beginners. In these syndromes, water is forced under high pressure into all sorts of nooks and crannies when the patient-to-be falls at high speed, or is towed in a sitting position. At best, such a tumble can leave you with an incredibly clean acromphalus.

The more ominous sequelae were reviewed in the *Annals of Emergency Medicine* in 1980 by Dr. Kenneth W. Kizer of Hawaii. He summarized cases of lacerations, infections, and general disruption of the delicate plumbing down there, all due to falls during waterskiing. Complications included miscarriage, infertility, and bleeding requiring surgery – sometimes on the driver of the boat.

Thus, we doctors recommend that anyone who either has a womb or has spent time in one avoid waterskiing at speeds faster than five miles per hour. Even safer, try standing on your waterskis in your bath, gripping your soap-on-a-rope firmly with both hands and making vroom-vroom noises with your mouth.

The Vicious Cycle

You can look it up.

In the last ten years, there has been a dramatic increase in the number of people riding ten-speed bicycles. Over the same period there has also been a steady increase in the number of people dying from cancer.

Coincidence? Perhaps; perhaps not. Doctors are ready to blame almost anything on bicycles – and with good reason. In recent years, several new neurological and urological complaints have been discovered among riders, syndromes that give new meaning to the expression 'the vicious cycle.'

One of the first of these diseases was dubbed 'Cyclist's Palsy' by Dr. Thomas A. Converse, a cyclist himself. He described 'an insidious onset of numbness, weakness, and loss of coordination in both hands,' a condition that soon left him unable to hold a pen. His illness turned out to be due to pressure on his palms from the handlebars leading to compression of the ulnar nerves – actually, a common problem among cyclists. Fortunately, this condition is responsive to several months of riding around in the back of a Daimler.

Since then, several other syndromes have tried to claim the title 'Cyclist's Palsy' for themselves. Most are blamed on the hard, narrow banana seat typical of ten-speeders – what urologists call 'Hell on Wheels.' These seats have been found to cause an inability to start urinating, an inability to stop urinating, inflammation of the prostate, and torsion (twisting a full three hundred and sixty degrees) of the testes.[1]

One forty-six year-old man, whose case was reported in a medical journal last year, lost sensation in his penis for one month after a bicycle trip, though he retained the capacity to become aroused and have intercourse. In short, he was able to have sex; he just didn't enjoy it. There's a philosophical lesson in that story somewhere and we hope you never learn it.

The Playing Fields of Eton

There will always be an England – at least if we heed the warnings of Dr. J. B. Bourke, a surgeon from Nottingham. Reprinted below in its entirety is his letter from the February 10, 1979 issue of *The Lancet*.

Gum Chewing At Cricket

Sirs, – The *Observer* of Jan 28 reported details of the injury to the Australian batsman Darling on the first day of the fifth test match in Adelaide. Darling was hit under the heart by an ordinary ball from Willis, collapsed, choked on his chewing gum, and somehow swallowed his tongue. When the crisis of choking was over, the injury to Darling was found not to be serious.

Over the past two or three summers whilst watching first-class cricket, I have noticed an increasing number of players chewing. On the second day of the Trent Bridge test match, at the beginning of the New Zealand innings, an urgent signal was sent to the England dressing-room and eventually the twelfth man brought out a packet of

---

1. Contrary to popular belief, enduring testicular torsion does not separate the men from the boys. Indeed, it tends to turn the former into the latter.

chewing gum which was quickly distributed among several players. During the two New Zealand innings, most England players were chewing and some replenished their gum, returning the tell-tale silver paper to their pockets. Subsequent inquiry revealed that chewing gum whilst playing first-class cricket is a common habit.

Chewing gum, inspired whilst playing cricket or other sports, may become lodged in one of the bronchi and cause wheezing or infection. If it gets stuck in the trachea, asphyxia and sudden death may ensue. The cricketer will be at greatest risk when he takes a sudden inspiration – as when hit in the abdomen or chest whilst batting (as in Darling's case) or when reaching for a high catch.

I am unaware of any catastrophe resulting from the use of gum by cricketers, but it is fortunate that skilled attention was immediately available for Darling – it will not be at most cricket matches. It would be prudent for cricketers to abandon this apparently widespread habit, and we must hope that youngsters will not follow the dangerous example now being set by English and Australian test cricketers.

J. B. Bourke

Scrum Pox

Since rugby, rather than soccer, tends to be the traditional winter sport for most English public schools, it's clear that the game will be thought a cut above most others. Anyone who comes through the public school system more or less whole in mind and body (about enough pupils for a XV) might well have become addicted to the business of rolling around in the mud with a bunch of sweaty men wearing shirts like David Hockney's.

The game's advantages are that once it's over you are

at liberty to drink gallons of beer, sing obscene songs, and throw up. After that you can apply for a job with a city brokerage firm. Among its disadvantages — apart from the usual fractured skulls and mashed spinal columns — is Scrum Pox, a condition that is beginning to reach epidemic proportions.

This syndrome is not a disease per se; it is a blanket term for skin infections transmitted during the face-to-face contact of scrums. According to a recent report in the British Medical Journal, the problem is limited to forwards. But among those players the problem is severe. One hospital team had seven cases among fifteen players in a recent season. A gentleman's agreement prevents these players from competing; but before big matches, this agreement, along with other vestiges of civilization, is routinely forgotten.

For years, the cause of scrum pox was obscure. Some thought it was a form of another skin disease associated with athletes known commonly as 'Jock Itch.' This notion was too disgusting to contemplate — even in prop forwards. Recently, microbiologists have isolated several different bacteria and viruses as the guilty agents. The most common of these may be a form of herpes virus that has been variably called herpes gladiatorum or herpes venatorum, (Latin: *venator*, sportsman. Impressed?).

This disclosure merely strengthens our conviction that rugby is a sport to be avoided. If one must get herpes, we can think of a better way. Still, this new data has spawned a variety of recommendations on how to avoid scrum pox if you insist on spending your Saturday afternoons with those big, sweaty boys:

1. Never wear tight or suggestive clothing.
2. Wear rubber gloves to receive passes.
3. Refuse to scrum down.
4. Stop washing your rugby strip. If there is inadvertent physical contact in the game, it won't be repeated.

5.   Never drink another player's beer after the game. You don't know where his moustache has been.

Slot Machine Tendinitis

Doctors who live or practice near casinos have long known of 'Slot Machine Tendinitis' – inflammation of the right shoulder resulting from repeated yanking of the one-armed bandits' arms. According to a medical journal report of May 28, 1981, steroid injections may help, though the best treatment remains rest or an early jackpot. If these fail, we recommend attacking the machines with a crowbar. In any case, if you can afford to play long enough to hurt the shoulder before the wallet, we don't have much sympathy for you.

Another article in the same journal described a related syndrome, called 'Space Invader's Wrist.' This disorder represents a strain of the ligaments used in the rapid, repetitive arm movements required to play the popular video game. It's a fine example of technology bringing its own exclusive afflictions.

Urban Cowboy Rhadomyolysis and Other Dangers of Dance

Disco and punk rock may well be the most important cultural developments in this country since commercial television but, from a medical perspective, they are choreographed stockcar races.

How else can one feel after learning of 'New Wave Subconjunctival Haemorrhage?' As recently described in *The New England Journal of Medicine*, this syndrome consists of bleeding in the whites of the eyes after doing the 'pogo' – a dance that involves little more and nothing less than jumping up and down for hours. It's difficult to have much sympathy for the victims, or for those who suffer from 'Disco Felon' – a hand infection resulting from repeated snapping of the fingers. Finally, there's the dread 'Urban Cowboy Rhabdomyolysis' –a massive destruction of muscles from riding mechanical bulls.

Of course, not all injuries are so exotic, as shown in a 'Survey of Roller Disco Dance Injuries' by Dr. Matthew Corcoran of St. Columcille's Hospital near Dublin, published in 1980 in the *Journal of the Irish Medical Association*. After a roller disco ballroom opened near his hospital in 1979, he kept track of all injuries treated in his emergency room that could be connected with this new form of dancing.

Over a one month period, the casualty list included twenty-eight victims. Half of them had broken bones, most commonly the wrist. Three required hospitalization and general anesthesia. The other patients were treated for lacerations and/or blunt trauma, and sent home.

By comparison, Belfast must have seemed safe.

The list goes on and on. We haven't the time or space to go into diseases like 'The Short Leg Syndrome' – an orthopedic disaster resulting from running in only one direction on a banked track. Its once-vigorous victims are consigned to a lifetime of Walter Brennan imitations.

Suffice it to say that sports doctors are working around the clock – well, several hours a week, anyway – to understand the physiology of complaints like 'Tennis Eye,' (in which a well-hit tennis ball travelling at more than fifty miles per hour can cause serious damage to your eye) or 'Sports Sunburn.'

What you do with this data is your business; only later does it become ours. In the meantime, we will try to be compassionate, though it is difficult to sympathize with many patients, especially the runners. While we have heard of the concept of running through pain, we cannot understand why anyone would want to do such a thing. Running *away* from pain makes so much more sense. Thus, we advise that when playing any sport you keep constant vigilance for any sign of discomfort. When pain appears on the horizon, stop immediately and take a taxi home. Examine yourself, pour yourself a drink. And tune in to *Grandstand*.

5
How to recognize your own psychiatric emergencies

'Doctor, am I going crazy?'

This question, so often unspoken, dominates many of the encounters between patient and doctor. All too often, the patient goes home with his doubts unresolved, believing that his doctor might be uninterested in his mental health, and so reluctant to raise the issue.

Not necessarily! True, most of us in the medical profession consider mental illness an ugly business and spend a good part of our day hoping the topic won't come up. But, when dealing with the anxious patient, the doctor is usually groping for a way to broach the subject himself. Even when he does not directly raise the question, he may offer subtle signs that it has crossed his mind – the arched eyebrow, for example, or sudden snorts of laughter. He may leave his stethoscope in his pocket throughout the exam. Or he may not examine you at all, but write a valium prescription after only a few minutes, while murmuring something about 'medicine for your muscle spasms.'

What can this mean? Are you really crazy after all? Experts agree that, more often than not, the answer is yes.

For proof, psychiatrists cite the famous Mid-town report on the prevalence of psychological disorders in New York City. Psychiatrists felt that 81.5 percent of those surveyed were 'less than well,' while 23.4 percent were considered 'impaired.' True, the era was the 1960s, and all the participants lived within walking distance of Bloomingdales. Taking these factors into account, it has been estimated that the actual 'impaired' rate is no more than five percent in the general population. Among our readers, of course, the figure is closer to 87 or 88 percent.

So what to do? Can you afford nine years of analysis just to discover that you're nuts?

The solution is self-treatment, using time-honoured (and relatively cheap) outlets such as compulsive overeating, knuckle-cracking, and stuttering. Professional psychotherapy should be reserved for those times when all hope is lost anyway.

Of course, successful self-treatment demands the ability to recognize crises when they are upon you. Which brings us to the point of this chapter – how to recognize your own psychiatric emergencies.

Now you may read parts of this chapter and think you recognize yourself. Do not panic. If you suddenly realize that your constipation is consistent with psychotic depression, there's little to be gained tonight by looking in the Yellow Pages under 'Shock Treatments.'

Go to the refrigerator. Take a bite out of everything in sight. Then read on. You may have something much worse.

Depression

We all have periods when we are overcome by sadness or sensations of helplessness and insecurity. These feelings are not normal. They add up to the syndrome of depression – what we doctors call 'The Blues.' Clinically, this syndrome can range from mild adjustment reactions, such as often follow the death of a loved one, to severe psychotic breaks, like those routinely seen in Latin America after the home team loses a football match.

There are several drugs useful in cases of depression, but experts agree that the safest and most effective method for many patients is electroconvulsive therapy – better known as shock treatment. Unfortunately, given the world-wide energy problems and our current quest for independence from Arab oil, we cannot oblige everyone in need of a good dose of blue bolts. For example, the electricity demands of Liverpool alone after an Everton away win in a derby game would require the construction of two nuclear reactors. As it is, even those lucky few sick enough to get treatment receive only a fraction of the voltage we would like to give them.

The problem, then, is calculating just where on the spectrum of depression you lie, and how badly you need treatment.

Mildly depressed people are usually acutely aware of their loneliness. They solicit aid from friends, and look for magical solutions to their problems. They frequently imagine that regaining a lost love or winning an idealized new one will instantly reverse their fortunes. A fine portrayal of a mildly depressed man was offered by Robert DeNiro as the homicidal Vietnam veteran in *Taxi Driver*.

In cases of severe depression, people often give up. They do not look to their friends for hope or relief. They are sure that others cannot or will not help them, and that things will never improve. Unfortunately, they are usually right.

Confusion arises over cases of 'masked depression' – when the patient protects himself from feelings of sadness by simply denying that they exist. Other clues are usually available, however, and good psychiatrists can recognize them, gain insight into the patient's defences, and tear them apart. Gradually, the patient learns just how profoundly depressed he really is; and occasionally this insight is the deciding factor in an unconscious weighing of the merits of suicide.

For example, depressed people commonly manifest their absorption in themselves with unusual concern for their physical health. They may be certain that they have a cancer or fatal infection – a punishment that, at some level, they are certain they deserve. They wander from doctor to doctor in search of confirmation. If you know anyone who fits that description you should immediately buy him a copy of this book.

In recent years, however, as appreciation of the complex interactions between body and mind has increased, depression has been shown to be associated with actual physiological changes. Doctors use these clues to diagnose depression, and so can you. For example, the metabolic rate of such patients often slows and many gain weight. Alternatively, appetite may decrease and they may lose weight. Some patients cannot fall asleep; others sleep constantly. Another common complaint is conspitation, though early depression can be marked by diarrhoea.

These pointers ought to help to eliminate confusion from the mind of any rational person.

Anxiety Attacks

Anxiety attacks are common, relatively minor psychiatric emergencies that are often characterized by the sudden onset of shortness of breath, a feeling of tightness in the chest, nausea, a cold sweat, and a tingling sensation around the mouth and fingertips.

These spells are especially important because they must be differentiated from heart attacks, which often begin with shortness of breath, chest tightness, nausea, a cold sweat, and an unusual sensation in the arms and jaw.

One quick way to make the distinction yourself is to breathe into a paper bag. (Never use a plastic bag. As every mother knows, if you even look at a dry cleaner's bag when alone in a room, it will wrap itself around your face and suffocate you.)

If you are having an anxiety attrack, rebreathing your own carbon dioxide will correct a blood disturbance that is increasing your drive to breathe. The sensation of shortness of breath will pass, and the attack will break. (Burt Reynolds used this technique in the film *Starting Over*, and twenty minutes later he was in bed with Candice Bergen.) Of course, if you are having a myocardial infarction, your heart needs every atom of oxygen it can get, and breathing into any kind of bag could kill you.

If you do go to a casualty department, we suggest going to one where you are not yet well-known, or, perhaps, go wearing a simple disguise. This single precaution will give a true heart attack a fighting chance of getting diagnosed. By considering the history, the examination, the electrocardiogram, and the results of some blood tests, the doctor will decide which diagnosis is correct. If you are having an anxiety attack, he will reassure you, tell you to get some rest, and give you some Valium.

In contrast, if you are having a heart attack you will receive the most advanced care medicine can provide. You will be rushed into a coronary care unit, a great many blood tests will be drawn, and rather large needles will be stuck into your arms or some even less convenient part of your anatomy. You will be hooked up to a cardiac monitor while being examined by several doctors and perhaps even a medical student.

Then you will be reassured, told to rest in bed, and, to keep you as calm as possible, you will probably get some Valium.

Dementia

'Doctor, am I demented?'

In surgeries across the county, doctors face this half-question, half-plea, over and over every day — occasionally several times within fifteen minutes from the same patient. Usually there has been trouble at home. Maybe the patient has heard his children joke about his 'toys in the attic.' Perhaps he has noticed that, in little ways, he is slipping. Some days he may wake up in the wardrobe. On others, he may get to the lavatory and forget why he went there. Before long, the demented patient says little and does even less — all to avoid embarrassment, until he can confront his doctor and try to get an answer.

We have a simple way of dealing with this question. We pretend we didn't hear it. If, after a few minutes, the patient appears to have forgotten the question, we say 'Yes.' Since the patient doesn't know what we are referring to, no one's feelings are hurt.

For these unfortunate patients, dementia becomes a way of life. To doctors, though, dementia is a distinct clinical syndrome. Usually it is irreversible; many cases are due to arteries getting plugged up by cholesterol plaques — the penalty of a lifetime of fried-egg sandwiches and high-tar cigarettes. As blood-flow to the brain slows to a trickle, the neurons decide to pack up and call it a day.

Other people have an inherited tendency to suffer the premature death of brain cells. Researchers do not fully understand how the damage occurs; nor can they state the likelihood that any given person will become prematurely senile. Still, if your father began to laugh pointlessly or chew on his tie while still in his fifties, you'd best get your affairs in order now.

There are, however, a small percentage of cases in which a treatable cause can be found. Among these causes are thyroid disease, infections, and nutritional disorders such as pellagra and vitamin B–12 deficiency. Thus, it is important for the physician and the patient to remember that dementia means disease and to recognize its early signs.

No sign is as important as memory impairment. Demented patients are fully alert, and often have excellent long term memory – that is, they can remember details of their childhoods with startling clarity. Their problems lie in constructing new, short-term memories. For example, they have trouble with the names of new people and places. They may even forget things they have just heard or read!

Many patients first note that they have difficulty with calculations. They may be unable to understand how much money they owe the grocer, and how much change to expect. To cover themselves, they simply hand the assistant a £10 note, and accept whatever change is returned. This strategy has never endeared old people to newspaper sellers and, as inflation runs wild, it is becoming less effective.

Other patients initially notice the cardinal complaint of dementia – memory impairment. Demented patients are fully alert, and often have excellent long term memory – that is, they can remember details of their childhoods with startling clarity. Their problems lie in constructing new, short-term memories. For example, they have trouble with the names of new people and places. They may even forget things they have just heard or read!

Another serious problem for the demented is handling abstract ideas and broad philosophical concepts. They are often forced to retreat to safer ground, rigidly holding to familiar slogans like Hegel's postulate that reason is the conscious certainty of all reality. Meanwhile, they are tinting their hair blue in order to keep it from turning yellow.

All these problems become more severe when compounded by the most common manifestation of dementia – memory impairment. Demented patients are fully alert, and often have excellent long term memory – that is, they can remember details of their childhoods with startling clarity. Their problems lie in constructing new, short-term memories. For example, they have trouble with the names of new people and places. They may even forget things they have just heard or read!

Naturally, these deficits force demented people to retreat from society. Ironically, the rate at which dementia progresses will accelerate when someone is bereft of his social function, such as his job, or loses physical capabilities. In their isolation, many patients develop paranoid notions about others, or even about their own bodies. For these unfortunate types, too, this book would make a wonderful gift for Christmas, or just as an unexpected surprise.

Last but not least among the many features of dementia is memory impairment.

Remembering what has been forgotten is, of course, technically impossible, as pointed out by thinkers from Plato to Des O'Connor. After all, if something can be remembered, then it wasn't forgotten in the first place, was it? Thus many of you may have difficulty making the correct self-diagnosis.

One quick test is to ask yourself whether reading this section gave you a headache. If the answer to that question is no, then the answer to the question posed at the outset – whatever it was – is yes.

There are several remedies to the problem, none wholly satisfactory. If you are in an occupation such as politics, you can go on for some time before being found out and appointed ambassador to Spain. Jobs demanding more skill, such as being shot out of a cannon at the circus, may require major adjustments in your life.

One approach some of our patients enjoy is to leave your spouse, take up with someone younger than your children, and bequeath him or her all your money. If that doesn't turn things around, we recommend going to discos to remind yourself that, bad as life is, there are others who are much worse off. In any case, there's no point in fighting. Go with the flow, knowing that at last you can say or do anything you want without anyone raising an eyebrow.

Neuroses

Patients constantly ask us whether we think they are neurotic. Usually, we are successful in stifling retorts like, 'Is the Pope Catholic?' Stealing a line from our psychiatric colleagues, we come back with 'Why do you ask?' Not as clever, perhaps, but it does let them talk.

Through this technique, we have learned that the most crippling neurosis among the post-war generation is one we call 'The Fat Child Syndrome.' This syndrome is epidemic among those born in an era of peace, prosperity, and – above all – plenty. Raised on butter instead of guns, they thought being worldly meant eating French toast and Danish bacon.

Not surprisingly, a lot of them got fat. Today, many have slimmed down, but remain psychologically scarred by too many trips to the outsize department in clothes shops. They are left with a disturbance of body-image reminiscent of schizophrenia. Even when not on a diet, they feel that they are breaking one. Guilt and fat have been internalized.

Answering a few quick questions can help you assess whether you are neurotic about your weight, and suffer from the Fat Child Syundrome:

1.   When you were a child and your parents offered to buy you a pet, did you ask for a dog but secretly want a tapeworm?
2.   Do you weigh yourself:
     a. Every day.
     b. Naked.
     c. After going to the loo.

d. After running several miles and letting the sweat dry.
   e. All of the above.
3. Do you despise your skinny brother who weighs himself once a year, fully dressed, holding a book, without even emptying his pockets, and in public places like railway stations?
4. Is your wardrobe devoid of horizontal stripes, because back in 1962 your mother told you that horizontal stripes made you look even fatter?
5. When people tell you that they can't believe you were ever fat, because you look so thin now, is your reaction to distrust them?

If the answer to any of these questions was yes, then probably the answer to all of them was yes. Doctors are very sympathetic to victims of the Fat Child Syndrome, since it is so common among doctors themselves. When we were kids, and our friends were out playing football, we were inside getting smart and eating Mars bars.

As is true for most neuroses, there is no cure for the Fat Child Syndrome. We recommend staying away from rich puddings and rugby shirts, and not bringing any progeny into the world.

Paranoia

Being paranoid isn't as much fun as it seems from the outside. After all, paranoid people are loners. They collect injustices. Vivid memories of minor slights are never forgotten. They get inappropriately angry waiting in queues, in heavy traffic, or when jostled in a crowd. They take it very personally when they get arrested.

Predominant, of course, is a suspiciousness that stems more from insecurity than any real danger. Paranoid patients are constantly looking for hidden meanings and secret motives in any gestures. A minor incident can remind them, at a subconscious level, of some vulnerability apparent only to themselves and they will respond with wild rage in an attempt to compensate. These attacks of rage are normal, and even useful when driving in London, but they can poison human interactions such as business negotiations or getting second dates.

Having been through a lot of the former to get the latter, we are especially pleased to reveal that a treatment for paranoia finally exists. This medical breakthrough can eradicate any irrational fears lurking in your soul and put you at peace with the world. But we are not going to provide you with any details because we want to hurt you.

Obsessive-Compulsive

The obsessive patient, who often appears to be so effective with the details of daily life is, in reality, caught up in a continual conflict between obedience and defiance. The question he constantly asks himself is 'Shall I be good, or shall I be naughty?' What distinguishes him from the rest of us is that he briefly considers being good.

The roots of this conflict generally lie in the early power struggle between parent and child, a struggle that often focusses on bowel habits – specifically, toilet training. Some psychiatrists feel that early toilet training – say, before the age of two – may push a child toward an obsessive personality, while letting the child find his own way in and out of the lavatory will result in a more normal development. Other experts say that those psychiatrists have been paid off by the manufacturers of Pampers and rubber sheets.

Nevertheless, they *do* agree that life is a joyless endeavour for these patients. They tend to be preoccupied with dirt, time and money, as well as with squeezing their toothpaste from the bottom of the tube. Answering a few quick questions can help you decide whether you are among them:

1. Did you get upset when you learned that the sun is a middle-aged star?
2. Do you worry about the affect of continental drift on property values?
3. Is your idea of a good time picking your teeth?
4. When Faye Dunaway was scrubbing the floor in *Mommie Dearest* did you get enthusiastic about it? (Be honest.)
5. It's eleven o'clock. Do you know where your children are?

If the answer to any of these questions was 'yes', then you are an obsessive-compulsive type. The prognosis is grim. You will probably never know the emotional intimacy of a close relationship. If you think you have had one in the past, think again — it wasn't so great, was it?

But don't worry — you can have something even better. Head for the nearest medical school and make your way to the admissions office. Offer your neatly typed name in application. You may never be truly happy, but it sounds like you will make a terrific doctor.

Schizophrenia

Schizophrenia is the most complex of psychiatric disorders, and if you were expecting us to straighten this mess here, you have made the common error of confusing this book with *An Elementary Textbook of Psychoanalysis* by Charles Brenner M.D. Too late now. Let's just say that schizophrenia involves much more than 'split personalities.' And if you feel that there are eighteen people inside you, and three or four are stable enough to hold down a decent job, you've got off lightly.

Schizophrenia is a disturbance of several areas of psychological functioning. Many patients have trouble defining their 'ego boundaries.' This term does not refer to fighting in the Wimbledon dressing-rooms. It involves the inability of the patient to determine where he ends and another begins. This means he cannot tell if thoughts are yours or his. If someone speaks, he cannot be sure he didn't do the talking. Sometimes, he can't even tell whether an arm or leg belong to him or someone else. It's like being in a rush-hour tube-train all day long.

Not surprisingly, the schizophrenic patient has difficulty organizing his thoughts by the usual rules of logic. The border between illusion and reality is lost. Words or gestures take on unintended meanings, often sexual or paranoid. Notions of which patients are ashamed take on the form of disembodied voices.

As a convenient test to determine whether you are an evolving schizophrenic, we have prepared the following set of questions. What have you got to lose in answering them? It's already been a long night. Turn the light on, and respond with a firm 'yes' or 'no.' Equivocation will result in government surveillance of a V.A.T. inspection.

1. Do you hear voices in airports?
2. Do you really think that if you put ten pence in that machine you will be able to get a chocolate bar out?
3. When Michael Foot fell asleep during the last Party Conference, did you agree with his Press Secretary that he was only pretending to doze to see if Tony Benn would try anything?
4. Do you believe that if a dog sleeps on his back, he's gay?
5. Do you own a Sony Walkman?

If the answer to any of these is 'yes', you are an impending schizophrenic. You should feel lucky to be British. As a schizophrenic, you will become eligible to break just about every law in the book and still have people defend you. This land was made for you and me.

Though material in this chapter has covered the principal disorders of mood and thought, we realize that, like many tracts written by doctors for the layman, it skirts key issues. Rather than deal with the concrete problems of everyday life, it falls back on what is known in the trade as 'Psychiatric Mumbo-Jumbo.' The reader may not understand how this data is relevant to his or her life. Well, in short, it's not dirty enough.

Do not despair. For now, and only now, you are prepared for the thorniest difficulties in the life of the anxious — an area of medicine so closely bound with psychiatric emergencies that usually the most the doctor can do is try to work out which came first. We are speaking, of course, of the subject of the next chapter — Sexual Dysfunction.

6
The hypochondriac's guide to sexual dysfunction

In recent years, sex has made its way out of the changing room and into the doctor's surgery. Everyone agrees that the shower floors are a lot less slippery as a result, but medicine has been complicated immeasurably. Most doctors would nevertheless concede that the transition was inevitable, if painful. After all, sex is not a game — it is an incurable disease, or at least the most powerful invitation to human suffering we know of apart from medical college. Hippocrates himself thought that sex might one day be a medical concern, and he warned doctors to be ready. 'Sooner or later,' he said, 'this entire mess is going to fall into our laps.'

He was right. Today, sex is the doctor's problem. The change was more sociological than medical. The sexual revolution that began so innocently two generations ago with the TV show 'Muffin the Mule', eventually swept the country, even destabilizing parts of Scotland. It produced radical changes in values. Sexual fulfillment became the name of the game, the toast of the town, the heart of the darkness.

Unfortunately, you can put all the sexually-fulfilled people in Britain under the clock at Waterloo Station, and still have room for the Lithuanian Air Force Band. Which brings us to the point of this chapter – as revolutions go, this one produced more than its share of casualties. Doctors' surgeries are filled with the walking wounded. Much of our time is spent trying to decide which among them can be saved.

Despite this huge need, most doctors remain deliberately aloof from the whole issue – the principal reason that we felt compelled to include this chapter in *The Hypochondriac's Handbook*. Our reluctance to grapple with these complaints is puzzling to most patients. They expect doctors, of all people, to be able to deal with the problem of sex, free from the usual burdens of shame, ignorance, plague and famine. This apparent indifference should not be taken as evidence of a true lack of interest or compassion; rather it reflects the discomfort felt by most medical men when confronted by such matters — a discomfort that is often accompanied by mild nausea, fainting spells, and nosebleeds. For this reason, they will go to extremes to keep the topic even from coming up. Many of our colleagues will only see a patient if his mother or priest is present. Some set off their beepers and leave the room as soon as the subject is broached. Others immediately send patients for expensive tests: the more invasive, the better.

Some insight into the making of a doctor can clear up this mystery. By the time they are born, most doctors are too old for sex as we imagine it. At each step in his education, the doctor responds to the calls of unbridled passion by making safe, sublimating detours, maintaining a professional calm and a compulsive meticulousness to avoid scuffing his Gucci shoes. As a student in college, he watches the birth of tadpoles and then follows them through the miracle of the life-cycles as they become beautiful, drowned butterflies. This linkage of sex and death is reinforced by his observations of fatal allergic reactions in guinea pigs, which can turn blue and still maintain erections. (It's not as easy as it looks.)

As a tired houseman, he gets slapped around by nurses who have received formal training in fogging his glasses and shortening his stethoscope with a minimum of wasted motion. Finally, after years of sacrifice and the establishment of a successful private practice, the mature doctor can experience the ultimate sensual thrill of squeezing a Mercedes into a tight parking place, followed by hitting a golf ball cleanly while surrounded by people of the same colour as himself. No wonder he's not anxious to have the subject of sex come up.

In contrast, patients begin with a more natural attitude. As children, they possess a fearless enthusiasm for their bodies, as well as a pro-fessionally-gratifying desire to play doctor. Puberty —all too often dismissed as one more hair-raising experience — increases the stakes considerably, as heavy weather gear is checked out for use throughout life or until the age of fifty-four, whichever comes first. Unlike your socks, you *can* take it with you when you die.

Unfortunately, in the course of growing up and cultivating mature relationships, many people lose their child-like innocence and become alienated from the normal expression of sexual desires. The smallest of traumas can pull the plug in the sexual sink. A woman may suddenly feel unwanted when she sees her husband turn immediately to the bra section of the new mail-order catalogue. A man may discover that the secret words that arouse woman are 'American Express'. Both sexes may feel unable to live up to the unrealistic, stereotypic expectations about sexual stamina and accomplishment that pervade our culture.

So, by the time the adult reaches our offices, he regards sex as a physical and emotional vacuum. Like nature, he abhors a vacuum, yet is concomitantly compelled to rush into it. As far as he is concerned, a person's organs should never be seen and only occasionally heard from – any muttering from any tissues usually suggests, to the active imagination at least, imminent self-destruction. The sexual organs, however, are not common, everyday tissue. If inadequate attention is paid to them, they tend to generate their own publicity. If the patient tries to pretend that they don't exist, orifices that formerly dared not whisper their names soon refuse to stop shouting. In no time at all, the sexually-unfulfilled patient can be rendered completely incapable of concentrating on the more important issues of life, like renewing one's driving licence or practising a firm handshake.

Faced with a rebellious body and indifferent doctors, many patients try to ignore the rich animal and vegetable kingdoms that comprise the ratatouille we call sex. They wade upstream against the surging juices of their forebears, until every natural instinct is killed. The medical term for these unfortunates is 'Stockbrokers.'

We tell our patients that they should go with the reproductive flow! They should learn to recognize their own desires, no matter how bizarre. And if one of yours involves building a wooden box, you had better read the next section very carefully.

Koro

If a man walked into your office with his penis clamped inside a wooden box, what would you think? Being an ignorant layman, you would probably assume that he was collecting for charity and drop in some small change. Doctors wouldn't put any money in at all. We would know instantly that this man was a victim of Koro – one of the most curious manifestations found beneath the setting sun of sexual dysfunction.

This syndrome was first described by the British in

Malaysia,[1] but has been found throughout the world. A man with Koro syndrome suffers the delusion that his penis is shrinking, and that if it disappears inside his abdomen he will die.[2] Those afflicted with this delusion usually adopt the solution of tying a ribbon around their reproductive organs or, alternatively, encasing both kit and caboodle in a gaily decorated wooden box – a tactic we feel is especially hazardous to the caboodles. Such patients can develop subsequent medical problems ranging from splinters to premature jogging fatigue as a result of increased wind resistance.

Therapy for such patients can be very difficult. Doctors used to try to reassure sufferers that if, by chance, the penis should disappear into the abdomen, they certainly wouldn't die. We generally found ourselves conceding, however, that they would be better off dead. As a result, they would go out and build bigger boxes and burglar-proof them. Our own approach has been simply to make sure that the box conforms to the local housing standards and advise the patient to wear a table cloth instead of underpants. After that, we let the chips fall where they may.

Couvade

Couvade is derived from a Basque word meaning to 'sit upon eggs.'[3] It is an extraordinarily common condition in which men develop the symptoms of pregnancy, often to their amazement.[4] It's victims are always the husbands of expectant mothers, men who develop one complaint after another until they are suffering from

---

1. Only recently has a team of Malaysian anthropologists been permitted to enter England. We await their findings.
2. The premise may be faulty, but you have to give credit to the forceful logic of the conclusion.
3. As far as we know, this is the only word ever derived from Basque.
4. Not to mention that of their mothers.

severe morning sickness, headache, backache, and progressive abdominal swelling.

The pains of Couvade have no basis in physical diseases. They arise solely from hysterical imitation – a psychological demand for equal attention. Couvade has attained its full flowering with one African tribe whose men, at the appropriate time, take to the only bed in the hut and start complaining of labour pains. As the rest of the village, including the shaman or witch doctor, gather around to help, sympathize and soothe, the pregnant wife goes off into the woods and has the baby. She returns, and kicks everyone out of the house and her husband out of bed, while the whole village rejoices to see him back on his feet.

This syndrome is also well-known in the West. The manifestations, though, are usually more subtle in this country. An early clue that one of our patients is about to have a difficult few months, is the discovery that he is wearing underpants with the logo 'Baby under Construction' stitched across the front. Such cases of Couvade can be difficult to treat. Fortunately, they tend to resolve spontaneously in about nine months, unless the patient is a male elephant, in which case a cure can take up to two years.

A doctor confronted with such a patient can take the easy way out. He can deride him, make jokes about his rhythm method, give the patient a dummy and play a tape of 'Where Will the Baby's Dimple Be?' over the waiting room intercom as the patient leaves the surgery. Or doctors could follow our example in recognizing that this confused man needs help like any other patient. We attempt to reassure him concerning his symptoms, prescribe extra vitamins, enroll him in breathing classes and if the couple are private patients, charge them for two deliveries.

Pure Erotomania

We do not wish to imply that psycho-sexual disturbances are an exclusively male domain. Far from it. Take, for example, De Clarambault's Syndrome, popularly known as Pure Erotomania. Most reports of this disorder come from French and Italian literature,[1] but it is seen often enough in this country for doctors to realize that it is more than a psychiatic oxymoron – for many, it is a way of life.

The victims of this disease are usually, but not always, women. They become consumed with the delusion that someone is passionately in love with them. The 'lover' is generally a public figure who knows the erotomaniac only casually if at all. Still, once the notion has taken root it can dominate the lives of both.

Typically, the patient pursues her beloved relentlessly, waiting for the release of the passion she is sure she recognises. She follows him home, leaps out unexpectedly and embraces him in public, and sends sexually-explicit singing telegrams to him at work. These tactics never worked for us in college and are no more successful in these situations.

The patient's own marriage and children are abandoned as she seeks the presence of her beloved. He in turn often has some explaining of his own to do to save *his* marriage, as women with Pure Erotomania have been known to force their way through windows and into their quarries' homes. This can result in fascinating family dinners. Children develop better eating habits because they can't bear to leave the table during such encounters.

We have treated several such patients after trying ineffectually to get them to transfer their affection to ourselves. Some of our cases are already described in the medical literature, but we cannot write about them

---

1. Where else?

here without compromising the sacred doctor-patient relationship and the confidentiality of the medical record. We can, however, offer a composite case history based on the stories of three patients who, to protect anonymity, we can only refer to as a doe-eyed newscaster, a former Wimbledon champion and an Iron Lady.

A young woman, 'Miss D,'[1] fell hopelessly in love with a Member of Parliament while working in his Central Party Office. Though quite pretty, she was socially his inferior; unable to read or write, her only accomplishment had been winning a beauty contest sponsored in her home town by a leading manufacturer of flea collars. The MP ('H'), on the other hand, had been given the freedom of the city of Milton Keynes and was one of only a handful of Shadow Cabinet members who called the party leader 'Mike.'[2] He was cool to her advances, until she discovered some photographs while ironing old correspondence. Then they got married.

Within a short time, the MP died after catching Lassa Fever from a troop of Nigerian Girl Guides ('N') who had flown over to take part in a Day of Action rally. His wife inherited his vast fortune, including natural gas deposits located on his Scottish estate ('S'). She went on to become a member of the board of directors of one of Britain's leading hotel chains.

This pathetic case history indicates just how persistent the delusory state can be. The cost in human lives and laddered tights is incalculable. Attempts at treatment can be very frustrating for the concerned practitioner because of the duration and depth of the neurotic delusion. Ultimately a more or less permanent stay in hospital or confinement to the Isle of Eigg may be

---

1. Not her real name.
2. He also called Shirley Williams, George Brown, Geoffrey Howe and everyone else 'Mike', but that's another disease for another chapter.

necessary to prevent the patient from harrassing her 'lover' or extracting her revenge.

Piblokto

Piblokto is not truly a disease of sexual dysfunction. It is included in this chapter because its victims are often mistaken for exhibitionists or Pure Erotomaniacs, and because we had no where else to put it. In truth, erotic thoughts are the furthest things from the minds of these unfortunate women.

Also known as the Arctic Hysteria Syndrome, Piblokto is an altered state of consciousness seen in Eskimo women who are fed up to their mukluks. They are tired of igloos, of huskies that can't be house-broken, of husbands who go out hunting, but end up trapping and skinning Ind Coope party-packs. For these women, being cold has lost its charm.

An otherwise trivial incident – such as being attacked by a wolf – can be the club that kills the baby seal. Once the Piblokto Syndrome is triggered, the victim pulls off all her clothes and runs naked among the ice floes, screaming gibberish. Gibberish, of course, shares certain linguistic qualities with normal Eskimo talk – the gutteral 'A', for example, or the tendency to spit when pronouncing consonants. This unfortunate coincidence has caused more than one Eskimo Maidenform woman to be institutionalized.

The attack passes after one to three hours. After-wards, the patient is completely normal, except that she will not remember the episode – in contrast to her neighbours, who usually can't forget.

This sort of attack represents a rejection of the patient's situation in life. It is an extravagance which allows the patient to butter her bread on both sides in the nude. It permits the discharge of built-up emo-tional steam rather than turning it against oneself. The patient is, in fact, better able to maintain a normal life after the release of her hostility.

This syndrome is only rarely seen in Britain south of the Outer Hebrides, where television game shows provide a similar outlet for the ritualistic discharge of aggression.

Priapism

Though our discussion thus far has emphasized the psychological, doctors know that when it comes to sexual dysfunction, there is more than one way to run over a dog. No matter what your analyst told you, there is a physical side to sex. Of course, disorders affecting the tools of the trade are inevitably less varied than the disturbances created by a fevered imagination. Cruelly enough, though, they tend to affect men more than women and have therefore received a lot of attention from both doctors and Rotarians. Perhaps the cruellest of all is priapism.

Priapism refers to a persistent erection of the penis[1] — persistent to a troublesome degree. Contrary to the popular myth, the name is not derived from General Nho Gho Priap, the Korean explorer credited with discovering the prostate. Actually, it is named after the Roman god Priapus, who invented the concept of the tradesman's entrance.

This condition is almost always harmless, if embarrassing, but it can be due to tumours of the bladder or prostate. Although one might reasonably conclude that all adolescent males between thirteen and eighteen are in the process of being consumed by bladder growths, such problems are quite rare. Most often, psychological disturbance leads the patient up the slippery slope of priapism. These conditions are disgusting, and we refuse to discuss them further.

---

1. Or limb, as it is referred to by our grandmothers.

Impotence

Doctors are rarely troubled by the emotionally debilitating, uncontrollable erections of priapism. There is less and less of that sort of thing as one moves up in years and tax-brackets. Sexual arousal is considered to be a sign of poor breeding.

In contrast, impotence can lead to no breeding at all – an example of what William Blake called a 'fearful symmetry,' and what one woman we know described as 'a crying shame.' Which points up one of the most crippling features of this problem – like bad breath, impotence is usually called to your attention by someone else. Not surprisingly, the complications that follow all too often extend beyond the bedroom. With impotence comes the stigma of failure, a lack of vigour, an inability to make snap decisions, or a tendency to snap one's decisions too quickly.

The causes of this complex complaint are numerous and they are reviewed every few weeks by certain magazines. In most cases in which an etiology can be determined, the problem is psychological. Fear of failure, fear of women, fear of appearing vulnerable, fear of cutting yourself, and fear of your mother discovering those magazines top the list. Alternatively, you could have cancer or diabetes.

Even if you have, the great problem for you and other impotentates is understanding that impotence is not necessarily a problem at all. Your gun may be spiked for sound ecological reasons.

As scientists from Malthus to James Burke have pointed out, our greatest long range danger is too many people. Nature has devised many ways to control overpopulation among other species. If there are too many lemmings, they run into the sea and drown. If there are too many caterpillars, they eat all the leaves and die. If there are too many stray dogs, someone orders them rounded up and shot.

But Nature has considerably more difficulty with

human beings, especially those subpopulations that are the greatest drain on our resources (advertising executives and civil servants.) Humans don't like to swim out too far. They won't eat most leaves because of terrifying experiences with their mothers. Warfare was a good idea, but too nonselective. It tends to remove those most beneficial to society, as in the case of Ted Williams, who was plucked from the Chelsea forward-line in 1942 after scoring twenty-eight goals that season, including three hat-tricks.

Impotence is the alternative to war, the most conscientious of objections and the most passive of resistances. It is a phenomenon unique to human beings.[1] It may be Nature's way of letting us out of this mess with a whimper, not a bang.

Fatal and Near-Fatal Allergic Reactions to You-Know-What

The characters: You and the man of your dreams.
The place: Yours or his, it doesn't matter.
The context: Deep affection, genuine mutual respect, shared interests, all adding up to true love, both spiritual and physical. At the moment, mostly physical, as you are in bed, making love.

After an appropriate period (we recommend two or three minutes) you feel your heart beating faster — pounding against your chest. Your breathing becomes rapid and shallow. Gasps and tiny strangling noises emerge from somewhere at the back of your throat. A

---

1. We are so confident of this assertion that we issue a standing challenge. If you can find one impotent animal, we will send you a free copy of this book. Send us two impotent animals, and we will send you two books. Get the idea? Simply post the animals in a box with holes so they can breathe, to the British Medical Association offices.

tingling sensation spreads over your arms and legs. Your skin becomes pink, then mottled. You feel your head throbbing: the room starts to spin.

You may be having an orgasm. Big deal. Alternatively, you could be having a severe allergic reaction to your lover's semen and the next breath you take may be your last. It's difficult to tell.

For years, doctors did not believe that this syndrome existed and dismissed case-reports with remarks like 'What a way to go!' But researchers have now shown that some women really are allergic to proteins in the semen of their lovers. Exposure can trigger a massive allergic reaction, as if one were experiencing the world's largest bee-sting. With appropriate medical care almost all survive, though victims tend to be a little gun-shy in the future.

If you suspect that you may be allergic to someone's semen, multiple allergy shots will not help. We recommend keeping a loaded syringe of epinephrine under your pillow. This drug has many actions, including making the heart work much harder, but it will reverse most severe allergic reactions. Be careful not to inject your lover, or the earth may stop moving for him for good.

In preparation for sex, carefully arrange by your bedside a snake-bite kit, a bee-sting kit, a hayfever mask, a medical inhaler, and a pollen counter. You never know what else might be going around.

After considering these diseases and our reactions to them, one cannot help but feel that somehow mankind has lost its way. The rest of the animal world has an approach to sex that is mature, simple, almost casual. Admittedly, extreme tendencies exist in some species such as an inclination to devour one's spouse if one is not concentrating. Still, the few politician-like behaviour patterns of the animal world are more than compensated for by nature's decision to relegate sex to a few annual days of hysteria, with the rest of the year devoted to eating bark, making strange noises and so forth.

Do animals discuss senile impotence or jaccuzi climaxes with Russell Harty? Do animals wear underpants that say, 'I Can't Help It, I'm Italian.'? Do animals go out and buy extracts of sweat glands from dead rodents so they can get live ones to pay for dinner and a drink at my place afterwards? Do animals read (or write) articles like 'The Gnu You: A 53-Year Plan to Give More Style to Your Bounce and Make You More Attractive to the Pepsi Generation'?

No.

On virtually all other counts, man and animal think alike. They share the same fundamental desires for food, drink, loose shoes, and nice neighbours. Sex, and sex alone, defines the uniqueness of the human race. Carnal knowledge has alienated us from the rest of the natural world, and the chances that the natural world will take us back diminish with each passing day.

7
How to get into hospital

Getting into hospital does not carry the prestige of, say getting into Oxford. Indeed, to the casual observer, there are drawbacks to hospitals that make even four years in a Midlands polytechnic look reasonable. For example, a private room in a hospital makes a suite at Claridges seem like chicken-feed.

Still, the discerning patient understands quite well why getting into hospital can be so much harder than getting into a university, especially if you don't have the connections. Hospitals, after all, do so much more for the soul. For example, few colleges will send a clergyman to your room; in hospitals, they come without your asking. If you want drugs at St. Andrews, you have to go to the library; in hospitals, nubile young women bring them to you as you lie in bed. At the University of Sussex, you have to go to the lavatory; in hospitals, your lavatory comes to you.

Not surprisingly, we all feel a nameless attraction to the hospital and its emergency department. We go to the hospital because it is there, because the lights are on and someone must be up, because the doctor's surgery is closed and it's too early to go to the all-night chemist and see what's new in laxatives. We are driven by the same majestic and mysterious drive that impels a salmon to abandon its friends, leave the ocean, and swim upstream to the site of its birth – we were born there, we must return there, we might meet some girls there.

With shocking regularity, though, the would-be patient is turned away at the door, his complaint deemed too trivial for admission – an experience every bit as humiliating as getting those thin envelopes in April. Thus he learns that you can't gain admission to a hospital for a tune-up at your convenience. All too often, the way is barred by hostile nurses and sleepy doctors ready to tell you to take your anxiety attack and shove it.

It doesn't seem fair. You pay your NHS contributions. You don't litter much. You'd hire a handicapped person if a really attractive one came along. Why shouldn't you have as many medical tests as you want whenever you want them? 'We re-took the Falklands Dr. Schreiner,' you moan. 'Why can't you put me into hospital:'

Well, we can. We have devised an approach that has been highly successful in gaining admission for even the most timid of patients. Unlike alternative plans, our does not require that you should be double-jointed, carry BUPA cards, or be able to hold your breath and lie really still. If you can remember the phrase 'Professional misconduct' you have the talent to get admitted to any hospital at any time, sleep all day, eat custard out of little tins, and take drugs even the Pope can't get simply by asking for them.

The first principle of our plan is to resist the temptation to go to academic teaching hospitals in order to make your admission more prestigious. This error makes the admissions process much more complicated despite the fact that doctors there are very susceptible to hints of rare diseases, which can seem an advantage. Mention a family history of Grahmann's Syndrome, which involves mysterious fevers with periodic psychotic episodes, obesity, and underdeveloped gonads, and watch the entire staff mobilize. The tests ordered after admission are especially comprehensive if the disease to be excluded is extraordinarily exotic. They will cause many curious sensations, and may make you glow in the dark.

Unfortunately, patients using this technique run the constant risk of detection and severe punishment. At many academic institutions, for example, exposed malingerers have to eat their hospital dinner twice. At U.C.H. they are forced to see a different medical student each day, sometimes two — a brutal but entirely legal form of interrogation that has been known to empty entire wards.

So when you are just looking to get away from it all, we recommend choosing a local general hospital. Some of our patients have passed on helpful hints on how to pick the right one. Look out for a hospital situated on a lonely stretch of road near an old house high on a windswept hill. If the hospital sign is in blinking neon, with a Coca-Cola or Watney's logo, you're on the right track. The nurse may collect your wallet, rings and car keys before the doctor has seen you. This development means that you are about to be admitted or about to be robbed, maybe both.[1] If the doctor requires an interpreter to ask you whether you've taken out medical insurance, you've found your new home.

In the accident and emergency department, you should complain of a common ailment that cannot be quickly diagnosed. We are going to tell you about three such syndromes: those that cannot be ruled out in the emergency department. Each requires that you be admitted to hospital for observation. Each differs regarding the tests and drugs you will get. Your choice will depend on the mood you are in, your religious

---

1. If they take your belt and shoelaces, however, think seriously about leaving. And don't do your bird imitations to relieve the tedium of sitting in the waiting room. You're only asking for trouble.

whims, and whether you've been thrown out of that hospital before. For example, if you are neurotic about having sharp objects stuck in your back, then number three – meningitis – may not be for you. That's why we'll begin with the prototype of all complaints, the people's choice, chest pain.

Chest Pain

For millions of Britons each year, 'chest pain' is the magical phrase that opens the doors and parts the red tape. Not surprisingly, it is also the password for sophisticated patients everywhere. They know that many of the tests for myocardial infarctions do not turn positive for hours or even days, and that some heart attacks never show up on tests at all.

They also know that most doctors have heard of cases in which a patient, usually a friend of the powerful, came to the casualty department complaining of a vague discomfort. The patient was reassured that it was indigestion and sent out, only to die several hours later while trying to fill his prescription for Rennies. Such cases are called 'instructive' by doctors – that is, they teach us to write illegibly. Within the legal profession these tragedies are known as 'own-goals.'

So if you come to the casualty department complaining of chest pain, the doctors will try to determine if it is related to the heart. If there's any doubt, you will be admitted to a nice quiet intensive care unit bed where you will get mood-altering drugs and be allowed to rest. If you play your cards right, you can be there a week.

First and foremost, you need the right story. You must tell the first person you see that you are having chest pains. Many of our patients add the adjective 'crushing', but others think it a cliché. In any case, those words will immediately get you wheeled into a special room, while other patients who have lesser problems like pneumonia and knife wounds look on jealously from the waiting area.

In will come the houseman. He is apt to be irritated and a bit skeptical after a night of treating students who have consumed a bottle of vitamin pills in a suicide gesture. He'll be ready to flatten any hysteric who wanders into his cage, so your next few words and actions are crucial. You must look anxious and repeatedly mutter that you think you're going to die. Tell him that the last time you had this nameless dread was when you were in the front-line in Korea (younger patients could make this the assault-craft off Port Stanley). Breaking into a cold sweat is a nice touch.

The houseman will usually sneer and ask you if the pain is sharp, or burning, or worse when you take a deep breath. These questions are all ploys to write your pain off as coming from the lungs or stomach – anywhere but the heart. Breathing rapidly and rolling your eyes, you must reply that the pain isn't sharp, that it's more like a pressure in the middle of your chest. Now is the time to play your trump card. Your knitted brow should suddenly clear in an expression of enlightenment. Make a fist, clutch it to your breast, and wail 'IT FEELS LIKE AN ELEPHANT IS STANDING ON MY CHEST!'[1] Passing out briefly at this juncture will often help drive the point home.

By now, you will have the doctor's complete attention. He will know that he has a serious problem on his hands. To make conversation while he dries his palms, he may ask you how you feel. Tell him you feel like you want to throw up – rarely a good sign in medicine. Don't mention that what is nauseating you is the fear of explaining yourself to the police after insisting on an ambulance ride, and then being booted

---

1. This complex is known as the Levine Sign, after the famous Harvard cardiologist Samuel Levine. It is considered unreliable in Africa and India, where trauma victims will say 'I feel like I'm having a heart-attack.' – Hannibal's Sign.

out of the emergency department as a malingerer.

The houseman will then ask you about cardiac 'risk factors' — the conditions that have been found to increase the likelihood that a patient has heart disease. The strongest of these are:

1. Obesity.
2. Diabetes.
3. High blood pressure.
4. A family history of heart disease.
5. Smoking.

Obesity is hard to fake. So is diabetes, though it won't hurt to say that you don't think you have it, but your parents, your four grandparents, each of your siblings and the family St. Bernard all did, and you've never been checked.

At this point, ask if it is all right to light a cigarette with all the oxygen around. Explain that you usually smoke eighty to a hundred a day, but fewer than that when the coughing gets so bad you can't hold a cigarette between your lips or when taking a deep breath causes more blood to appear in your phlegm. He may say no.

Continue with your story anyway. Tell him you aren't positive about the diabetes, because you never knew your family all that well. You never had the chance. After all, you explain, both your parents died of heart attacks in their early thirties and none of your brothers or sisters survived to graduate from their school, St. Jude's Academy for Cardiac Cripples.

You might mention that you were kicked off the St. Jude's chess team for hypertension, but that you never had it treated. Why not? Well, the only trouble it ever gave you was an occasional nose bleed and spells of blurred vision.

By now the houseman will be getting a little nervous and may want to examine you. He will check your cardiogram (an electrical tracing of your heart beat that can tell doctors how your heart is working and detect your most secret thoughts) and take your blood pressure. Thrashing around, perhaps faking a convulsion, will effectively keep him from finding out that both are normal. He will listen to your chest with his stethoscope, searching for the murmurs, thumps, and whimpers that the heart makes when it is scared — when there is nowhere to run, nowhere to hide. Quietly humming every third note of the Leningrad Symphony may simulate these noises convincingly, unless he is a concertgoer.

In all likelihood, your exam and cardiogram are going to be normal. Here the gossamer links of trust that you've worked so hard to create will snap if you don't take the initiative. Tell him that the pain is starting to shoot into your jaw and left arm. This news will make him review the cardiogram and perhaps go for help.

He will return with a junior hospital doctor and together they may try the Levine Test. This little manoeuvre involves rubbing a spot on your neck over the carotid artery while asking whether the pain is getting worse. A neurological reflex will make your heart slow down and if you are having true heart pain the ache may diminish. Those who are not having heart pain, but desperately want to please, will say that, yes, the pain is getting worse. The doctors will respond by ripping off the sheets and showing the sheepish patient the door. To avoid an ugly confrontation, we recommend pausing and saying in a puzzled voice, 'This may sound crazy, but I think the pain is actually getting better . . .' If one of the doctors tries to repeat the Levine Test by wrapping both hands around your windpipe and squeezing, he may be on to you. Usually, though, they will know that they are beaten.

The houseman will prepare for your admission to the coronary care unit. He may ask you whether you are still having chest pain. Nod vigorously. (Not too vigorously). You will then experience the happy surprise caused by morphine percolating from your veins to the frontal lobes of your brain.

The doctors will check every few minutes to see if your pain has abated. As long as you can muster a grimace, the morphine will flow. The opiates will induce a sense of well-being and bonhomie, not to mention the sudden conviction that with one deft short-cut you have attained the ecstatic centre of the spiritual universe. Your ability to convey sincere pain, finely-honed after a lifetime of mental self-abuse, may be blunted. More likely, though, you will do as your father did during your conception and drift off into a happy sleep, unclouded by thoughts of tomorrow's consequences.

Appendicitis

Many patients suffer from the delusion that having appendicitis is the work of children. Doctors, though, know that children are busy enough with chicken-pox, school and learning how to smoke. Most children simply do not have time to have an appendix out; they survive into adulthood with these time bombs intact and ticking.

What is appendicitis? To answer this question, one must first ask what is the appendix and, as far as we can tell, no one really knows. The best medicine can do is describe it as a wormlike pocket that hangs just off the end of the large bowel. It's usually just a matter of time until it gets plugged up and inflamed, and then performs its only known function – paying for some surgeon's golf-clubs.

We offer this explanation to our patients with appendicitis who ask about their disease – 'Part of your body has turned on you and is attacking you from within.' They are rarely surprised, and this perspective helps prepare them for surgery.

As a way of getting into hospital, appendicitis has its drawbacks. Chief among them are that a virtuoso performance is rewarded with a knife in the side. Beyond that, there's little chance for an encore, no matter how thoroughly the symptoms are mastered. Finally, you don't get any morphine until after the operation.

Still, behind every cloud is a hospital bed, and patients who have had their chest pains debunked should not be afraid to come back with an ache below the belt. Giving a good story is easy. The manifestations of appendicitis are so varied that surgeons will listen to almost any complaint – pain, hiccups, horrid age spots – and say, 'That's consistent with appendicitis. Get the operating room ready.' Once the operation is under way and a normal appendix has been found, the surgeon will be forced to vouch for your story out of embarrassment – more than one doctor has prepared an appendix for the pathology lab by dropping the specimen on the floor and stepping on it. When all is said and done, you'll be left with a nice scar to show on evenings out with someone special.

The key, then, is selling the surgeon on the idea. Though we have pointed out that he will often accept a pretty lame story, it's courteous to provide a classic presentation. Tell him the problem began with an ache around the navel, but then the pain became much sharper and moved down and to the right. Many patients say the pain gives them an urge to move their bowels, or pass wind, but it would probably be a bad idea to do either while the surgeon is there. You'll want him rested for the operation.

If you're a private patient he will base his decision of whether to operate on both the physical examination and the result of his tax assessment. During the exam, he will be looking for evidence that the lining of the abdominal wall has become inflamed. Patients with appendicitis keep their abdomens rigid as boards, and demonstrate what doctors call 'rebound tenderness' – that is, when we press down with our hands and then abruptly take them away, the patient jumps in pain.

(It's even more fun than it sounds.) Extra points are awarded if the patient dislodges a ceiling tile.

If rebound is present, most surgeons will take you to the operating theatre. Their motto, after all, is *ubi dubitas, ex flagellatum*. (When in doubt, whip it out.) On the other hand, if your surgeon checks for rebound by bouncing you off the floor, you may want to try another hospital.

The surgery is brief and complications rare. In a couple of days, you'll be sitting up, plucking at that string on your hospital gown and calling for more pain killers. While recovering, do not despair that you only had one appendix and now it is gone, never to get you into a hospital again. Look at matters philosophically and remember that that is why God gave us the gall bladder.

Viral Meningitis

Our third syndrome offers an attractive alternative to having someone with hairy arms muck around inside your abdomen. It also beats trying to sleep in a coronary care unit amidst the background-roar of beeping machines and cardiac arrests. Finally, since it is contagious, this ailment will also discourage your doctors from bothering you more than once a day.

The disease is, of course, viral meningitis. It is a benign illness caused by a viral infection of the meninges, the covering of the brain. While you are ill, the key symptom is severe headache, much worse than the sort used for emergency birth-control. Like birth-control, however, it is associated with a mild degree of drowsiness and confusion. If these states are not dramatically different from your normal way of life, you may want to add sore throat, nausea, stiffness of the neck and convulsions.

Viral meningitis clears over several days without treatment other than pain killers; full recovery is the rule. The danger lies not in the disease, but in its similarity to the early stages of other, more serious infections that can inflame the brain and eventually cool the cortex. Meningitis caused by bacteria, for example, can leave your brain on a permanent rinse-cycle if not treated promptly. Either syphilis or tuberculosis can cause similar symptoms. (People who cough at the wrong moment have been known to end up with both at the same time.) Thus doctors are often obliged to admit patients with viral meningitis for observations until these less pleasant illnesses are ruled out.

So come in complaining of a stiff neck, severe headache and sore throat. Wear a pair of underpants on your head, talk wildly of Shirley Thatcher and throw up on the doctor's shoe. Have a convulsion. (Remember that real convulsions are followed by several minutes of profound weakness and confusion. Bouncing up and asking, 'How was that?' is not going to help your case.)

The chances are that you will be admitted for several days of observation and a few simple tests. For example, they may take an X-ray of your head which, when framed, makes an inexpensive personal Christmas present for your parents. More ominously, though, you will have to undergo a spinal tap. A spinal tap is a procedure that involves inserting a needle through your back into the base of the spine in order to sample the fluid that bathes the brain and spinal cord. It's like drilling for oil, except that hitting a pocket of natural gas is not so much a cause for celebration as a reminder that doctors can be sued for malpractice.

The spinal tap is performed with you sitting or lying on your side with your back exposed to the doctor, who is holding the needle, and a nurse who is holding the doctor. During the course of the tap, you will probably hear the six most commonly used lies in medicine:

1.   I've done this a million times.
2.   This won't hurt a bit.

3. Here's a little bee sting.
4. The worst is over now.
5. We're almost done.
6. Now that wasn't so bad, was it?

If a medical student is also present, you may overhear a number of technical comments during the procedure, including:

1. Thanks for letting me try it. This is great. I feel like a real doctor.
2. Does spinal fluid usually smell this bad?
3. Where is all the blood coming from?
4. Have you ever seen anything like this before?
5. I can't get it out. Should we call the surgeon?
6. Jesus Christ!

Which brings up a rather painful issue. Sometimes the challenge of getting in to hospital is exceeded only by the challenge of surviving what happens once you're there. After a while, searching tests and powerful drugs can lose their charm. So it's likely that after several days of breakfast and bathroom in bed, when the heart attack has been ruled out, the appendix whipped out and the spinal fluid drained out, you will be ready to make a bid for freedom. And, in fact, matters usually resolve themselves satisfactorily; patients leave feeling refreshed and ready to take on their medicine cabinets.

But not always . . . Unfortunately, it is remarkably easy to get sick in the hospital, particularly if you have been under the supervision of a doctor rather than, say, an orderly. Medicine, after all, is not an exact science, but an art. Each test, each treatment, represents a calculated risk. Every doctor who is honest with himself knows that he has learned some lessons from mistakes; that's why we call our work 'practice.'

So if you have been in the hospital for far longer than you expected, if you have been in so long that your hospital number was moved to a dead-files system, it may be time for you to make the first move. Cancel your BUPA or PPP subscription and tell the hospital administrators that you have lost all your money by investing in Italian-Ethiopian war bonds. You will be shipped home by overnight mail.

8
Tissues and answers

Over the years, many patients have written to us, making the misguided assumpton that we write a popular health-advice column. Faithfully answering these letters in order to alleviate needless suffering has been an incredible nuisance. To forestall the expected avalanche of whining missives that will be the public's response to this book, we are publishing a list of the most common questions we hear, and our compassionate, medically informed answers.

Q. Over the past week, I have developed a runny nose, a slight temperature, and a cough that doesn't bring up much phlegm. My elderly father also has this same illness. Could it be cancer?
— N. N., Sutherland, Scotland

A. Could be.

Q. I am a chicken trainer, and two days ago I was scratched by one of my chickens while teaching it how to swim. Every time I pick at the scab, it bleeds a little. Should I be worried that it hasn't healed yet?
— T. B., Diss, Norfolk

A. Yes, it could be cancer.

Q. When I urinate after a heavy meal, I frequently notice foam in the toilet bowl. Is this cancer:

— P. R., Aylesbury, Bucks

A. Maybe.

Q. Can you settle a bet? My brother says that Japanese food carries tapeworms, and I say it is the cleanest food in the world. Who's right? The loser has to disembowel himself.

— E. H., Gerard St, London

A. So sorry, your brother is correct. Raw fish, a favourite in your country of origin, is often infested with a tapeworm called *Diphyllobothrium latum* (pronounced like the Welsh township). This parasite's eggs are carried by fish who swim where raw sewage is dumped and make the mistake of not holding their breath. Once the fish is cooked, the tapeworm eggs are no longer dangerous. However, cooks who sample lutefish or gelfilte as they are preparing them often become infected. In these and other patients the tapeworms can live up to twenty years, and grow to a length of twenty feet whilst causing problems like low blood counts, fatigue and the blues.

The best way to avoid tapeworms is to avoid fish from contaminated waters, and to cook all freshwater fish thoroughly. There is no foolproof way to determine which fish in the market are egg carriers, though several of our strangest patients have described methods of fish selection that have worked for them. We pass them on to you:

1. At the supermarket, pick up the prospective fish purchase and shake it vigorously near your ear. If you hear anything loose, put the fish down at once. Stick your fingers into powdered milk to kill any eggs that might have come off on your hands. If the supermarket manager starts giving you a hard time while you are

testing all the fish, tell him that your mind is being controlled by Barry Manilow and let your eyes mist over. He will leave you alone.

2. Place the prospective fish purchase to one side and stare straight ahead. If you see the fish making a movement out of the corner of your eye and it suddenly stops when you stare at it, there are tapeworms inside. Set the packet on fire immediately.

3. If you are unable to test the fish in the supermarket, take it home and place it on the kitchen table with a tape-recorder next to it. Turn the recorder on while making a coughing noise. Casually mention to no one in particular that you are going upstairs for a nap. Come back in fifteen minutes, take the recorder up to your room, and replay the tape. If you hear the tiny sounds of a bon voyage party with clinking glasses and shouted toasts, those little bastards are in there.

Q.   Catherine the Great. Did she die the way I think she did?

— J. Breeling, Kippax, Yorks.

A.   No, that was Nelson Rockefeller.

Q.   My little daughter gets hiccups all the time. It's affecting her marks at school, and driving us crazy at home. We're desperate. Can you help us?

— Y. Knott, Rickmansworth, Herts

A.   Your daughter should be seen by a doctor to rule out the presence of any diseases that can cause hiccups. (See 'Common Complaints'). Probably, none will be found, and your daughter will turn out to have either benign idiopathic hiccups that may pass with time, or else just plain bad manners. In either case, we recommend holding a pillow over her face for fifteen minutes. She won't have hiccups anymore, what's more her shoe size will never change again.

Q. I've heard a lot of stories, and I'm hoping you can set me straight. Will ... you know ... touching yourself make you blind or drive you crazy?
                    – O. Nan., I.O.W.

A. It's too soon to tell.

Q. Because my medical problems are so rare no M.D. can diagnose them, I've had to see a hundred and twenty-eight different doctors in the last year. Some of them try to rush me out of the surgery after only an hour or so, but I've found that faking a language barrier or congenital deafness can stretch most encounters into the better part of an afternoon.

Seeing lots of doctors for one visit each was fun while I was young, and it's a great way to stockpile Valium prescriptions for three-day weekends. But it's become boring. I think it must be psychologically destructive for me to have to start from scratch every time. I'm ready to settle down now with just one practitioner, and I want your help. How can I find Dr. Right?

                    – R. L., Birmingham, West Midlands

A. Your concern is completely appropriate. Choosing the right doctor is even more important than disinfecting the lavatory bowl. He's the one who is going to have to sign all those sick-notes. Without his cooperation your obsessions could result in the loss of your job, so he is bound to be a central figure in your life. In selecting yours, you should look for the right combination of credentials, credulity, and credit ratings. Some clues:

Take a look around when you are ushered into his surgery to await his arrival. Are there bars over the window? Is there a bar on the first floor? Are the free drug samples easily accessible so you can put them in your pocket without having to ask every time? Look for pictures of his children on his desk. Do they resemble game fish? Is there a picture of a wife in a family group or has someone placed a piece of black electrical tape over her face?

Is the language on his diploma in an alphabet you recognize? The further it is from Indo-European roots, the better off you are. Does his name end in a vowel or a grunt? Is his first name only two letters? Do the certificates on his wall include an award for Sunday School Attendance? Is it signed by a dictator?

When he comes in, look closely at him. Do his socks match? Do his eyes match? Is there evidence of superficial skin ulcerations? Does he breathe with his mouth open?

Tell him there is an officer from the Drugs Squad waiting in reception to talk to him. Observe whether he leaves by the door or window. While he's gone, examine his desk. Count how many stockbrokers and lawyers are listed in his address-book. Look for any listings under 'Parole Officer.' Are there prescription pads stamped with several different names? Look in his white coat for toys.

With these tips, you should be able to find the doctor who is right for you, together with enough incriminating evidence to keep him in line for years to come. These years will be filled with return visit after return visit. Yours will be a relationship richer than most marriages – full of themes, and beneath them, counter-themes. Underneath these, there will be counter-counter-themes. And underneath *those*, there will be bargain-basement prescriptions. Every visit will be anticipated for days in advance, and mulled over for days afterwards. By then it will be time to start anticipating your next appointment the next confrontation between two old and familiar rivals. Ali and Frazier. Spurs and West Ham. Dog and cat. You and your doctor.

Good luck to you, and remember that today is the last day of your life so far.

Q. Is it true that the government is trying to give us cancer by putting poison in tax forms that you inhale when filling them out?

— G. S., St. Helier, Jersey
(temporary address)

A. Could be.

Q. Are old people really interested in sex?

— K. C., Penzance, Cornwall

A. Yes, they are. The only problem is that they sometimes misplace it.

Q. I am worried about becoming infested with parasites. I am God fearing; I don't smoke or eat. I don't watch David Attenborough's programmes. I do not kiss anyone who is not British. What is a parasite anyway, and how do you catch them?

— G. B., Surbiton, Surrey

A. Parasites are dirty crawling things that are uglier than Arthur Scargill in a dress. They are the principle export of Chad, and are considered a delicacy in Libya, but nowhere else.

They are everywhere. They are found in dirt, under fingernails, over Luton, on walls, on barbers' combs, and in lawyers' briefs. Some parasites burrow into your skin, while others like to be inhaled. A few drift gently into your eyes as you sleep, while many are night deposits dropped into your blood stream by ambitious mosquitoes. There are parasites that live in your intestines, whose eggs can clog your liver like lemons in a lavatory. There are parasites that work in your blood cells and play in your brain.

Take Naeglaria. Please. This charmer is a germ that lives in lakes and swims up to your nose and into your brain. Another reason not to fall in when waterskiing.

These self-sufficient cells can do anything you do but better, especially multiply. They're pretty good at subtracting, too, if you catch our meaning. No one knows why they prefer renting to home-ownership, or even why they exist. Recent findings suggest that they were put on this earth by a vengeful God.

Q.   I love diet-drinks and, in fact, drink about twenty cans a day of my favourite brand. It's manufactured by a company that has its production-plant near Porton Down and they advertise it on TV as the lemon-lime drink that glows in the dark. I have to drink it quickly because otherwise it tends to eat through the sides of the can.

I say that if I buy it in a shop, then it must be safe. My boyfriend, who recently took out an insurance policy on me, thinks the stuff is dangerous, and that I will end up as a silhouette on *That's Life* making grunting noises while Esther Rantzen asks me if I am bitter over the loss of my ears. What do you think?

– S. Gharib, Salisbury, Wilts

A.   Our position has always been that almost anything in moderation is safe, and almost anything in excess is dangerous. Cut back to sixteen or seventeen cans a day, and keep checking your ears to make sure that they aren't getting loose.

Q.   I have been quite ill with Rocky Mountain Spotted Fever, which I caught while hunting endangered species near Aspen. I am recovered now, but I don't even remember having been on a mountain with spots. How could I have caught the disease?

– J. W., Leominster, Hereford

A.   You appear to have suffered a certain degree of brain damage as a result of your infection. The high temperatures can occasionally cause a premature thawing of your cerebral cereal. We appreciate the amount of effort it must have taken to write to us. As a gift, we are sending you a subscription to *Reader's Digest*. Stay at home, mix yourself in a glass of water, and read it. Don't write to us again.

Q. Is Slim Whitman a diet food?

> — J. W., Leominster, Hereford

A. We told you not to write to us again.

Q. I'm a twenty-three year-old blonde, and my friends tell me that I'm attractive. That doesn't have anything to do with what I'm writing about, but I bet it caught your attention. I want to know whether you think it is okay for doctors to call patients by their first names. My doctor does, and I'm not sure I like it. Is it all right for me to call him by *his* first name?

> — C. R., Leeds

A. Hippocrates, the first doctor to develop a knowing leer, used to say that patients could call him whatever they liked, as long as they didn't call him reverse-charge. Doctors have been using this same old joke ever since, though no one has been known to actually laugh at it.

We personally prefer to use formal terms when addressing (and especially undressing) patients. We feel that it is psychologically destructive to treat patients like children and thereby increase their sense of vulnerability. Calling patients by their first names, or 'dear' or 'sweetie' is a common error made by our colleagues. We consider such practices vestiges from the days when medicine was patronizing and sexist.[1]

---

1.   Nov. 14, 1952 to Dec. 2, 1953.

We believe that good medicine demands high standards of professionalism, ethics, and respect for the patient as a person. Thus we insist on calling all of our patients, no matter how attractive, buy their last names until at least the third or fourth date. It's a matter of principle.

Q. Will touching frogs give me warts?
– F. T., Tolland, Somerset

A. No, that comes from lustful thoughts.

Q. I am writing from a very nice hospital where I have been staying for three months with recurring bouts of chest pain that the doctors can't seem to understand. I am an old man with no family, and I like it here. The nurses think I am cute, and I get to wear my wellington boots in bed. It's fun to walk along with the back of my hospital gown open and not get arrested. Every morning, I get my favourite breakfast of eggs and morphine. I am worried that they are going to make me leave if they can't find something wrong. Do you have any suggestions?
– K. T., Bournemouth, Dorset

A. There is no single thing one can do to prevent getting ejected once the doctors think that there is nothing wrong with you. The most effective strategy for you is to slow the process of evaluation by stalling on every test or procedure that comes up. With luck, a routine admission can be stretched from days to months or even the better part of a decade.

A simple device for prolonging hospitalization is to knock over the receptacle that the nurses are using to collect the twenty-four hour urine samples the doctor has ordered. They will have to keep repeating it. If they schedule you for an X-ray of your stomach because of your constant complaint of abdominal pain, quickly swallow something from the other patients' lunch trays just before going down to the radiology department. They will either reschedule you, if you get caught, or diagnose a stomach-growth that resembles an Eccles cake. The tests that ensue will be exciting.

If these tactics fail, some of our patients recommend switching beds and identification bracelets with other patients – the MX Plan. Another strategy is to write notes in your own chart, pretending that you are a consultant. In your notes, express anger that certain tests have not been done, and request that all those completed be repeated. If nothing else works, you can always try dressing up like a junior houseman (unshaven, mismatched socks, stained tie, gummy stethoscope, a hundred and seventy pens). They will never let you leave.

Q.   I am only four feet tall, I stoop, my spine is covered with ulcerated lumps. My fingernails and toenails are chronically infected; they are thick, scaly, and smell like dead dogs. My complexion is beige with disfiguring blotches in harvest gold and avocado green. I can't bend any of the joints in my one leg. My drool has resulted in an unsightly fissure on my chin.

Why did God give me a body like this?
                                                              – S. K., Deptford.

A.   Why do fools fall in love?

Q.   I am one hundred and five years old. I have been in the hospital almost eight years this January. I came in to visit my sister and somehow got in the wrong queue. They took all my belongings, and gave me a pillowcase to wear. My bed has a view of a curtain (but a nice curtain). I have a large airy room which I share with twenty-five other girls. It's not too bad here. I like food, and I like my baths, and the noises at night remind me of my camping days when I was a Brownie.

What worries me is this: I don't know what's wrong with me, but I know it must be bad because every morning for the last five years, the nurses have greeted me by saying, 'Oh, what a pleasant surprise!' If I really am dying, I'd like to know it, because I'd like to discuss whether I want heroic measures like a respirator or PAP smear. Unfortunately, I haven't seen a doctor here since 1979. How can I tell whether I am slipping away, and what the doctors intend to do about it?

— R.I.P., Chingford, Essex

A. The question of whether to employ heroic measures for a terminally ill patient is a matter of the gravest importance, and should be discussed between the doctor and patient to ensure that the patient's wishes are respected. Sometimes, though, the doctor just forgets. It's difficult enough just trying to keep up with the changing rates of supertax.

Still, there are certain clues as to whether your doctor expects a Christmas card from you next year — clues that might help you decide about planting your garden with annuals or perennials. For example, getting a rosary with your All Bran breakfast can be a bad sign, as is the nurses' request for you to return your oxygen mask when you are finished. If your doctor leaves a brochure on group tours to Lourdes, you have a legitimate cause for concern. It's also worrisome if they move your bed closer to the lift, or if you find the nurses using your chest X-rays as placemats.

One final piece of advice to help with your investment plans: if more than ten percent of your body now rests in various biopsy jars, it would be best to stick with short-term deposits.

9
Examination of the self

The Examination of the Self is such a natural and essential part of a doctor's day, that we often forget that you don't know how to do it. However, we certainly understand your desire to learn. As this book has already shown, the danger from within is always present, and your body is less a vessel than a threat. Since most doctors examine patients only once a year, by the time an illness is detected it has often reached the stage we call 'Too Late.' So it's up to you to fill in the void between annual physicals with punishing self-scrutiny.

This reliance on Examination of the Self fits perfectly with the new militancy popular among patients today. They have assumed responsibility for their own health, though with more than a little ambivalence. The willingness to assume command of what seems a sinking ship follows a bitter realization – that they are prisoners within their own bodies, and that they have incommutable life sentences.[1] To make the best of a bleak situation, they have taken charge of their own bodies. And why not? No one else seems interested.

---

1.   See the best-selling treatise, *Our Bodies, Our Cells*.

Unfortunately, this duty often turns out to be more demanding than expected. Examining one's own body requires a sense of vigilance and awareness that adds new levels of meaning to the word 'introspection.' It also helps to have several mirrors on flexible handles. Most of our patients have instinctively devoted their lives to this task. They study their bodies with an attentiveness that is impossible to duplicate outside the autopsy room. The problem is that they don't know what to do with the data.

To the untrained observer, the body is a well oiled machine – but one that came without the instructions. Well-intentioned patients try to listen to their bodies with the intensity of musicians listening to a symphony – alert to every change of key, and to every broken string, not to mention the chewing-gum under the piano stool. All too often, however, they just don't understand what they hear.

It's embarrassing to admit, but doctors do a pretty shabby job of teaching patients what they need to know – a reflection of the general lack of interest in preventive medicine among the medical profession in this country. Indeed many doctors want nothing to do with the patient until something is clearly wrong. Unconsciously, they may even try to drive the 'healthy' patient away – especially if he is a frequent visitor. Some end sessions abruptly by announcing, 'see you next year. Get it? Next year!' Others stamp 'Do not open before Christmas' on the patient's chart as he looks on, or, better yet, simply toss it into the wastepaper basket. When these tactics fail, the doctor might try passing out during the examination explaining, upon regaining consciousness, that he has had this problem for months, that the spells are coming closer and closer together, and that he can't for the life of him work out what's wrong.

So we wanted this, the crowning chapter of *The Hypochondriac's Handbook*, to provide you with all the instruction you need to develop your own routine for a constant monitoring of your vital and not-so vital bodily functions. With the aid of this data, you should be able to scrutinize each tissue each day in the search for disease – a process we doctors call 'The Organ Recital.' Every morning, before pronouncing 'All Systems Go,' you will put yourself through a systematic checking, double-checking, and checking yet again that makes NASA's preparations for a moon-shot seem trivial. With any luck, you'll find something slightly amiss, abort your mission for the day, and head directly back to bed.

Where to begin? It has been said that your face is the mirror of your soul. (It has also been said that your face is uglier than a dead frog in a bowl of punch.) Finding something on it that everyone else already knows about but has been afraid to mention is no fun. Thus we urge our patients to begin their examinations with the head's various orifices – the ears, nose, and throat. If you have other orifices in your head, we don't want to know about them. We just had lunch.

Ear, Nose and Throat

No area of medicine is as baffling for the layman as the ear, nose and throat – abbreviated as ENT by patients, but called 'otorhino-laryngology' (rhymes with 'tremendous fee') by doctors. This sort of polysyllabic one-upmanship helps to keep the patient off-balance and remind him who's boss. One reason for bafflement, is that the anatomy up there is so complex: interconnecting tubes, spirals, and blind passages abound. If the whole mess wasn't so small and filled with mucus, it would be a great place to play 'Dungeons and Dragons.'

Instead the ear, nose and throat serve as a wonderland for children who are discovering their own bodies, and haven't reached the good parts yet. (See *The Hypochondriac's Guide to Sexual Dysfunction*.)

Events occur together that seem magically, if somewhat randomly, linked. They blow their noses, and suddenly they can't hear. They are eating lunch and someone makes them laugh; incredibly, milk shoots out of their noses. Their ears feel funny in a lift; they swallow, and all is well. Out of nothing, their bodies fashion lumps of wax and whatever. They ask their parents to account for these miracles, and they are told to go and watch television. In short, they learn for the first time that we do not live in a rational world.

As they grow older, go to school and mature, they learn to accept the body's idiosyncrasies and inside-jokes – even to laugh along as if they understood. They may never work out how that milk got into their noses, but after a while they stop asking why. There are, after all, adult otorhinolaryngological mysteries to ponder. For example, what is that tiny hunk of flesh hanging down in the back of your throat? (Answer: The uvula. Many adoescents worry about the small size of their uvulas. These unfortunates answer ads for creams and exercises guaranteed to increase the size of their uvulas and therefore their popularity. Such gimmicks simply do not work. Accept the remnant that nature gave you, and work on developing other aspects of your personality.)

Given the delicacy of these tissues, even routine maintenance is fraught with danger and doctors do little to defuse the problems. Tasks as simple as cleaning one's ears are made out to be work for neurosurgeons or priests, sometimes both. Doctors will tell you that if you use a Q-tip, you will jam wax into your brain's parietal lobes, after which your brain will leak fluid until it resembles dried dog food. But ask a doctor what he uses and why he has all those Bic pen tops lying around. He will immediately find an excuse to leave the room.

Not surprisingly, this area is a virtual breeding ground for bad news. Minor complaints like a runny nose can mean Lethal Midline Granuloma, leprosy or

116

syphillis, while seemingly subtle variations from the norm may spell disaster. Are your teeth too far apart? You could have a pituitary tumour that is making your jaw grow. Too much saliva? Someone might be poisoning you with arsenic. Too little saliva? You may have Sjogren's Syndrome in which your salivary glands race the rest of you across the River Styx.

Understanding the pathophysiology behind these diseases is beyond most laymen – we gave up after two years of medical school. Instead, we rely on two tried-and-tested all purpose remedies – anthihistamines and mulligatawny soup. One, or a combination of these, is effective in ninety percent of otorhinolaryngological emergencies.

Beyond that, we teach our patients a *functional* self-examination – that is, one that tests the functions of the ear, nose and throat. We suggest they warm up their tongues and throats by saying, 'Red leather, yellow leather' three times quickly, first normally, then while holding half a cup of flour in their mouths. If the flour comes out of any other orifices, see a specialist immediately.

We examine our own hearing by seeing how far we can hold the telephone receiver from our heads and still make out the gist of what the patient is calling about. Testing each ear individually is equally simple. While patients are talking to us in the surgery, we casually stick a finger in one ear, and then the other, and listen for a difference. You should be able to pick up many of the key words of the conversation with either ear, while simultaneously hearing a dull humming noise that specialists call 'The Ocean.' (For this test to be accurate, the same finger must be stuck in both ears.)

Similar techniques can be used on the nose to test your sense of smell, but at the request of our mothers, we won't go into them.

Your Eyeballs

An incredible number of patients come to us full of superstitions about the so-called relationship between deviant sexual behaviour and blindness. We sincerely hope that these stories are not true. Still, a great many other things can happen to your eyes, and almost none of them are good. Worst of all, most of these diseases begin with subtle signs that can be easily missed, especially if you're not able to see terribly well.

For example, how long has it been since you checked if your eyeballs stick out too far? *Exophthalmos* can mean an overactive thyroid.[1] (Do not worry about this diagnosis if you have no other manifestations of thyroid disease, such as restlessness, occasional palpitations, or insomnia.) Tears may mean infection, arsenic poisoning, or strong emotion, all of which are to be religiously avoided. Other diseases nibble away at the corners of your vision before going in for the kill. Consequently, we advise our patients to check every few hours on whether they can see things that lie off to the side.

For obvious reasons, then, you should constantly monitor changes in your visual acuity, and the function of the muscles that move the eyes. There's no need for weekly appointments with the opthalmologist when you can examine yourself every day by giving your eyes a 'stress test.'

We like to test our eyes on buses and in trains by trying to make out newsprint from three feet away — roughly the distance involved in reading over the shoulder of another passenger. To make sure that we are seeing each word correctly, we read the stories aloud. The paper's owner will usually let you know if you have made a mistake.

Yet another favourite testing technique we apply in hallways and lifts is reading the names on necklaces

---

1.   Except in Greece, where it is a popular pet's name.

that women often wear. If you need to get closer than six inches, you may be in trouble.

Whenever things get a little slow during surgery we test each eye independently by first closing one eye, and then the other. Sometimes this manoeuvre upsets elderly women who think that we are winking at them. Such notions evaporate during the next part of our calisthenics, when we test our *medial rectus* muscles — the muscles that turn the eyes inward — by crossing our eyes and producing a double image of the patient. We usually tire of this exercise quickly, and move on to the next phase, which is testing the *superior rectus* muscles — the muscles that turn the eyes upward — by pulling on our lower lids and looking up. If done correctly, you will look like a Greek statue and the patient will scream.

Lastly, we test the *lateral rectus* muscles, which turn the eyes to the sides, by turning both eyes outward at the same time. Once you have achieved this, you may feel a sudden, atavistic urge to hunt flying insects. This is a primitive reflex that should not be encouraged.

These exercises should ensure that your eye muscles are free of unsightly flab, and prevent the middle-aged bulge that makes most people over fifty look like frogs.

If you have problems with any of these exercises or tests, you should see a reputable optometrist[1], as you may need corrective lenses. These will make you look smarter and clink like champagne glasses when you kiss someone else who wears spectacles. Be warned, though, that they do have serious side effects and, if you are a male, you should be prepared for irreversible changes in your relationships with women.

Doctors have found that men who wear glasses spend half of their waking lives trying to avoid situations in which they might get slapped. They know that when they get slapped, they won't look rakish and

---

1. A reputable optometrist is one who does not make you remove your clothes for the examination.

119

even more attractive like a Bogart or a Gable. Their glasses go flying across the room. They get these ridiculous little cuts on the bridges of their noses. They have to figure out where their glasses landed by the sound and by squinting in the general direction of the woman's follow-through. When they do find their glasses, the frames won't sit straight on their faces anymore. The woman offers to pay to have them fixed. It's humiliating for everyone involved.

For this reason, few men who wear glasses get slapped more than once in their lives – and usually that's by their mothers, who don't really count. Instead, they develop a style with women reminiscent of the foreign policy of France – they sort of hang around the edges of the fray, hoping something good will fall into their laps.

Some men tire of living in fear of sudden violence followed by myopia. They buy spectacle-cords, of the sort worn by professional cricketers and science students. Others invest in contact lenses – a psychodynamic switch equal in significance to a sex change. Some even stop wearing corrective lenses altogether. They end up seeing less, but enjoying it more.

Obesity

Patients often ask how they can tell whether they are truly overweight or just have heavy bones. This question is more difficult than one might think. A nationally known insurance company published a famous set of tables that defined 'normal' body weight according to height, but it was so controversial that they could only get it printed on the backs of rulers. The Royal Air Force developed a different set of standards, taking into account age, degree of activity, and how fast you fall with a parachute. Other approaches, equally scientific, involve lean body mass, surface area of the body, and how long the elastic in your underpants lasts.

These aren't much help to the plump hypochondriac trying to go it alone. At what point, you ask yourself as you gaze into the mirror, should I start worrying about my weight?

Of course, if you are forced to gaze into two mirrors, the answer is pretty clear. But for the rest of you, we have developed a set of practical criteria that do not require special equipment or a medical degree, and can be answered in the privacy of your own home:

1. When you are sitting in a park, do children think you are a ride?
2. Can you hear echoes in your navel?
3. Do you have to travel by wide-bodied jet?
4. Are you sometimes used to show home-movies on?
5. Are you forced to obey motorway signs directing vehicles of a certain size to report to the next service-area?
6. Are you unable to remember the last time anyone would sit on a seesaw with you?
7. When you get on a bus, does it register 'Tilt' and refuse to give you your money back?

If the answer to any of these questions is 'yes', you are overweight and should start working on an anxiety reaction immediately. If your answer to all of them is 'yes', then go back to the chapter entitled 'Ten Diseases You Were Better Off Not Knowing About', and re-read the section on Prader-Willi Syndrome very carefully.

In any case, we recommend developing a weight-reduction programme that includes not only a carefully-planned diet, but meticulous attention to your weight itself and how it changes throughout the course of the day. For example, weighing yourself before and after meals, even when dining out, can give you a new perspective on just how much you are eating. Of course, most of these weight 'gains' are eliminated in the following hours by perspiring, blowing your nose, and throwing up. Weighing yourself before and after any of these can be extremely satisfying. Documenting such subtle shifts is not easy, however, and requires that you weigh yourself in *exactly* the same manner every time. Here is our routine:

1. Lock the door.
2. Disrobe.
3. Perform whatever bodily functions you can think of to make yourself lighter. (Don't make us go into them . . .)
4. Step on scales.
5. Step off scales.
6. See if the needle is advanced beyond zero.
7. It isn't. Try to calculate how much your glasses weigh.
8. Step on the scales again, this time leaning to the left and back. You are now one and one-half pounds lighter. Smile.
9. Weigh yourself again, leaning to the right and forward.
10. Worry.

Your Teeth

A few words about oral care – in fact, very few, because like most doctors, we know almost nothing about dentistry. What we do know is this – only bad things can happen in there and the worst of these usually take place around and during your regular visit to your dentist.

The physical pain is bad enough, especially when combined with the psychological distress provoked by emotion-laden terms like 'root canal,' 'periodontal scum,' and 'Trench Mouth.' What really hurts, though, is the shame – the disappointment so clearly etched on your dentist's face after he says, 'Open wide'; the accusations, so often unspoken;[1] the implications that you could have done better.

There are two ways of dealing with this uncomfortable situation. One is to come back with a quick retort, like 'What do you want me to do – kill myself?' Another is to try to limit your guilt-feelings by making good oral care a habit. It's really difficult to choose, but we recommend the latter course and suggest the following routine after each meal:

1. Brush your teeth.
2. Take dental floss out of medicine cabinet. Cut off a piece equal to your height multiplied by your waist size. This should suffice for your upper teeth.
3. Apply with sawing motion between teeth.
4. Wait for bleeding to stop. If it takes too long you may have leukemia.
5. Consider giving up. Imagine yourself with dentures.
6. Floss a few more teeth.
7. Decide that dentures won't be so bad.

Your Skin

Few parts of the body beg for self-examination as powerfully as the skin, yet it is often overlooked in the restless search for disease. Why do we ignore this marvellous substance which comes in so many sizes and colours, seals in freshness, and proffers little hairs everywhere you look? Think where we'd be without our skins – unemployed, for one thing.

Our research suggests that patients ignore the skin because of youthful trauma. Typically, during those delicate formative years when life-long neuroses are

---

1. Not often enough.

gathering strength, an adolescent brings some subtle blotch to his dermatologist. Anticipating cancer, perhaps a rare type that will be named after him, he is instead told that the disfiguration is disgusting and due to lust; then he's dismissed.

Still innocent, the teenager tries several more times; with a spot that refuses to heal, a hair that grows faster than the others, the mysterious scaling between his toes. Finally, the dermatologist gets exasperated, slaps him around, and refuses to see him again. Such treatment should surprise no one, as dermatologists are the most irritable of specialists. Anyone who flays warts for a living serves a dark and hungry god.

Scarred by this experience, the patient can develop such an aversion to dwelling on his dermis that he can't expound upon his skin condition(s) to his doctor(s). In extreme cases, he will stop picking at his scabs and fail to keep up his weekly charting of the diameter and colour of every mole on his body.

This fear not only denies the patient a profoundly satisfying experience, it invites disaster. For who knows when some little blemish you'd like to think is a hickey will turn out to be the first sign of Dego's Disease?

This rare syndrome, also known as malignant atrophic papulosis,[1] affects the entire body, but it usually holds its first surprise party on the skin. A pimple may appear and then transform into a pale depressed area with a red border, not unlike West Berlin. The lesions are innocent enough to the eye, but if observed microscopically, it would be apparent that a small blood vessel has closed itself off the surrounding tissue has died.

These dead areas eventually leave unsightly draining infections. That's the good news. The bad news is that the same process is going on throughout your body, causing strokes, heart attacks and other mis-

---

1. Now you know why we call it Dego's Disease.

chief. The most common culminating event is a sudden perforation of the intestines – a painful catastrophe, particularly if you are having dinner at the home of your boss.

What is the best way to guard against Dego's Disease, those horrid age spots, and other warnings that the end is near? Careful inspection of every square inch of skin after each meal is a start. Some areas may be difficult to examine directly. Polaroid snapshops of these regions will not only give you a good look, but will also provide you with a permanent record for your health care files. But for God's sake, lock the door first, okay?

The Lungs

The lungs are the largest organs in the body, and with good reason. They are essential to three of the hypochondriac's most vital bodily functions – coughing, wheezing and smoking. The respiratory tract has become even more important with the growing popularity of low-tar and filter cigarettes, for without superb lung function, meeting your minimum daily requirement (MDR) of nicotine is almost impossible.

Even if you don't smoke or live in Birmingham, the world is full of hazards for your lungs. Ignoring air pollution for a moment, we are almost all subjected to lung toxins at work every day. Cotton workers, for example, get a disease called Byssinosis, characterized by dyspnea (shortness of breath), chest tightness, coughing and wheezing. Typically, these symptoms are worse on the first day after a temporary absence – thus the phrase 'Monday Dyspnea' is often used to describe this disease. Variations on this theme are well-known in other occupations and to school children around the world.

Not even fresh country air turns out to be safe. Doctors have known for years about Farmer's Lung – a chronic lung disease caused by your body's reaction to air-borne material produced by mouldy hay. And recently, a new entity was described in the *Annals of Internal Medicine* called Dung Lung – not a Vietnamese diplomat, but a respiratory complication of exposure to you-know-what.

Fortunately, the capacity of the lungs to absorb nicotine, nitrous oxide, and other essential vitamins is roughly paralleled by their ability to handle oxygen. Thus you can monitor your own lung function with the few simple tests that can be performed at home, at work, or on your way to the doctor:

1.   Hold your breath for an entire visit to the lavatory in a Chinese restaurant.
2.   See if you can blow out all the candles on your child's birthday cake while he tries to think of a wish.
3.   While standing in a queue, try to make a woman's earrings sway by blowing on them. Then see how far you can run without stopping.

If you fail at any of these, we recommend taking up smokeless tobacco immediately.

The Heart

Most people are taught in school that the heart is a pump. Having studied this organ in detail, we find the notion of comparing the power source of the cardiovascular system to a woman's shoe ludicrous. The hemodynamics, the potential problems, the odour – all these are completely different. If the heart is analogous to anything fashioned from human hands, we'd have to say it is a time bomb.

Just as a bomb only has so many ticks on its timer, we feel the heart has only so many lub-dubs to give before planned obsolence has its way – 2,575,4000,000 to be exact. Skipping beats won't help. Thus, the examination of the heart should concentrate on accurate determination of the rate at which the heart is beating, and then slowing it down as much as possible.

You can calculate your own pulse rate by listening to your heart for one minute. If you do not have a stethoscope, build one of your own by cutting up the tubes that carry brake fluid in your car and gluing them to baked bean tins. Or you can just feel your own arteries pulsing at your wrist while watching the clock. If you get a rate of zero, either your watch is fast or you are dead. If you get a pulse of 90 or more, your heart is probably beating too fast and you should make it slow down at once.

Most people can only 'will' their hearts to slow by twenty or thirty beats per minute. For further reductions in heart rate designed to get as much time as possible out of your two and a half billion beats, we recommend the following measures:

1.   Avoid coffee, tea or cola.
2.   Avoid psychological stress.
3.   Sleep as much as possible, at least sixteen or seventeen hours a day.
4.   Never run. Walk as little as possible. Use cars or lifts whenever you can.
5.   No sex, unless you are married.
6.   Have your thyroid gland removed.

The Rest of the Body

Self examination of the organs that lie below the diaphragm is both unpleasant and dangerous – unpleasant because the names of most tissues down there recall dishes in Hungarian restaurants that you are afraid to order; dangerous because touching this general area on purpose can be construed as a misdemeanour in common law.

For these reasons we recommend testing these

organs indirectly by subjecting them to physiological stress. Of course, checking out each organ individually is an impractical waste of time. We have found that all systems can be simultaneously tested each morning by simply starting the day with a hearty Indian meal, washed down by a couple of bottles of strong lager.

We won't bore you with the science. Suffice it to say that the curry will test the integrity of your stomach wall, while the fats will put your pancreas into overdrive. Your liver will be stimulated to mass-produce gallstones, while your spleen will be tied up fighting infection. Your kidneys will be busy with the lager. Finally, your legs will get a good workout, as the stuffed parahta is immunologically rejected from your bowels as a foreign body.

You have now completed a comprehensive examination of yourself. Do it again. Depressing, isn't it? Now you know why doctors are so moody.

The next step is up to you. Why not make an appointment with your doctor and give him all your news? You could draw up an alphabetical list of your symptoms to demonstrate how efficient you are. Your doctor will certainly see you in a new light (assuming he agrees to see you at all).

In order to gain his complete confidence in your own diagnostic skills, you will have to make some attempt to speak his language. Too often, the specialist terminology employed by doctors – words like 'thrombolysis', 'angioplasty' and 'puke' – go right over the patient's head. In order to save face, the patient will leave the surgery in ignorance of his condition and his fate. Meanwhile, the doctor is chortling to his partner: 'Can you believe that? He didn't know he had Landouzy-Dejerine Disease! And he *still* doesn't know.'

If you can learn 'doctor-talk', you will not only gain your doctor's respect, you'll begin to share his values, his attitudes – maybe even a girlfriend or two. You can make a start by mastering the terms in the glossary that follows this chapter. Once fluent, you will be qualified to go anywhere and tell anyone anything. Just like a doctor.

Glossary

ABSCESS, n.
A collection of fluid, teeming with bacteria, toxins, and other agents hazardous to health; the body's version of Lake Erie.

ACHROMATURIA, n.
Colourless or nearly-colourless urine. This finding doesn't mean much, but its something to look forward to at weekends.

ACNE VULGARIS, n.
Inflammatory disease of the sebaceous glands and hair follicles of the skin. Once considered to be caused by bacteria, chocolate bars and other foods, including powdered mashed potato. Now understood to be due to impure thoughts and stealing money from your parents.

ACROMPHALUS, n.
Abnormal projection of the navel. Osler won the Nobel Prize in 1896 for demonstrating that if you press your finger precisely on the acromphalus, you will have many sons and your daughters will care for you in your old age.

ACUTE, adj.
Sudden, without warning, as in the onset of Lassa Fever, of the departure of the doctor who recognizes it.

AKINESIA, n.
Without kinesia.

ALBINO, n.
Pigment of the imagination.

AMAZIA, n.
Without mazia; the medical term for the lack of breast development in females; described by Hippocrates as a disease long before it became chic.

ANOPHORIA, n.
Tendency of one eye to drift upward; a syndrome that when witnessed makes children throw stones and gives adults motion-sickness; rarely seen in busy, successful executives.

APPENDIX, n.
Finger-like projection from the colon; the body's idea of a knock-knock joke.

ATAXIA, n.
Without a taxi.

ATROPHY, v.
Shrinking, wasting away of an organ with disuse, such as a limb's muscles after a fracture, or the intellect after a sit-com.

AUTOPSY, n.
Diagnostic procedure by which the hypochondriac hopes for vindication.

BACTERIA, n.
Really, really tiny micro-organisms. Doctors talk about them all the time but, frankly, we're not even sure they exist.

BILE, n.
Bitter alkaline secretion of the liver, thought by the ancients to cause irritability and virtually all other murderous instincts, which phenomena are now

understood to be induced by too much non-decaffeinated coffee.

BITTERLING TEST, n.
A real pregnancy test employed early in this century in which a Japanese fish resembling a carp was placed in two pints of fresh water with two teaspoons of a woman's urine. If the woman was pregnant, a tube-like structure protruded from the fish's belly and festivities or fisticuffs commenced, depending on the context. Though replaced by blood tests, many of which do not necessitate killing animals, the Bitterling test survives as a delightful party game that proves a real conversation piece. Party kits with fish and material for ten tests are available at a special price to buyers of this book.

BODO, n.
Germ found in stale urine; one reason why we always recommend getting it fresh.

BORBORYGMI, n.
The gurgling sounds made by the passage of wind through the intestines. Traditionally a source of social embarrassment, these noises are what the doctor listens for when he places his stethoscope on your stomach. Although this manoeuvre is useful as a source of comic relief after the tedium of feeling for the liver, some doctors have attempted to predict the patient's future by interpreting these sounds, a service that is available only in a few academic research centres.

BRACHYGNATHIA, n.
Abnormal shortness of the underjaw. People with this condition are often hereditary peers and are not to be trusted.

BULIMIA, n.
Hunger experienced shortly after a meal. See PROSTATE.

CACOGENICS, n.
Race degeneration resulting from the reproduction of inferior gene-pools. The most poignant modern examples of this phenomenon are evident in some Fourth Division football teams.

CACOSMIA, n.
A neurosis centering on imaginary foul odours; so common a complaint among our patients that we have been forced to keep a vase of dead laboratory animals in our waiting room to remind these whiners just how bad things *could* be.

CAFFEINE, n.
A stimulant found in coffee, cola and tea known to cause anxiety, palpitations, gastroinestinal distress, and insomnia; used by doctors only when real amphetamines are unavailable.

CAR SICKNESS, n.
Nausea initiated by the introduction of new models from British Leyland; occurs in annual epidemics.

CEREBELLUM, n.
Ante post-bellum and post ante-bellum.

CERVIX, n.
Anatomical term referring either to the opening of the uterus or to the bones of the neck – an unfortunate ambiguity that has resulted in several famous operating theatre errors.

CHEST PAIN, n.
The patient's trump card, his definitive demand for attention; analogous to your mother's threat to tell your father, your father's threat to tell your mother, your wife's threat to tell everyone, or Nigel Dempster's threat to tell no one at all.

CHOLESTEROL, n.
Fatty substance that renders food palatable; found in abundance in almost everything worth eating, plus Big Macs. Every Briton has a special place in his heart for this lipid compound – his coronary aterties.

CHRONIC, adj.
Describing a condition that will not go away, despite the doctor's best efforts; sometimes a disease, often a patient.

CLITORIS, n.
Mythological part of the female genitalia popularized by feminist writers and other troublemakers in the 1970s as the centre of female arousal. The 'clitoris' was alleged to be essential for orgasm, a function now known to be dependent instead on the acromphalus.

COLON, n.
The light at the end of the tunnel; an organ of splendid promise and disappointing performance.

CORTEX, n.
That portion of the human brain charged with game shows, commercials, feminine deodorants, *Cross-roads*, and self-service psychotherapy; although lacking arms, it is considered dangerous and is on Scotland Yard's 'most wanted' list.

CRAMP, n.
1. Painful spasm. 2. Japanese surgical device.

CYANOSIS, n.
Bluish hue to skin, usually reflecting poor oxygenation of the blood. A very grim prognostic sign, its name is derived from the Japanese word for 'goodbye.'

DEATH, n.
The final effort of the patient to embarrass his doctor publicly.

DIAGNOSIS, n.
Eponym attached to complaints by a doctor to convey the impression that he can actually do something about them.

DIE, v.
Doctors never say this word, partly because they have so many synonyms to choose from – e.g. expire, pass away, be taken, go to one's reward, turn up one's toes, go West, cross the Stygian ferry, fall off the twig, bite the dust, kick the bucket, go to Davy Jones's locker, feed the flowers, cool, croak, box, beam up.

DIGLOSSIA, n.
The anomaly of having two tongues. If both tongues are forked, you have a complete table-setting in your mouth.

DISINFECT, v.
To kill germs by physical or chemical means. Common disinfectants include chlorine, iodine, alcohol, sulphuric acid, napalm, formaldehyde, and Listerine. We personally favour tequilla, which not only sterilizes everything it touches or is breathed on but also bestows a warm glow of accomplishment, a lift to the feet and a steadiness to the hands, especially before surgery.

DOCTOR, n.
Member of a small group of almost perfect people charged with high duties and occasional misdemeanours; v. To adjust facts to account for a greater reality or need, as in income tax returns.

ECHOLALIA, n.
The involuntary, parrot-like repetition of words and phrases spoken by others, frequently associated with twitching and unusual eye movements; seen in catatonic schizophrenia and Government press briefings.

ECMESIA, n.
The intermittent inability to remember recent events, although the memory of events before and after may not be impaired. The syndrome is classically seen in early senility, but may also have an infectious origin, as suggested by the ecmesia epidemics that tend to follow a General Election.

ECSTROPHY, n.
The medical term for turning an organ inside out. While ecstrophy may be safely and easily accomplished in one's own backyard with organs such as the stomach, esophagus, or bladder, it is advisable to forgo attempting ecstrophy with organs such as the prostate or the kidneys unless accompanied by an expert skilled in handling such tissue.

EGOMANIAC, n.
Disturbed patient who will not stop talking about his problems. We refer all such patients directly to psychiatrists.

ELBOW, n.
The joint between the upper arm and the forearm. Look closely at that loose, spongy, wrinkled bag of skin around the elbow when the arm is straight. It is the ugliest part of your body. It makes us sick to even think about it.

EMETIC, n.
Agent that can induce vomiting. See ELBOW.

ERUCTATION, n.
The act of belching; signal from a rugby prop forward that a meal is over or a romance has begun.

ETHER, n.
The first anesthesia, replaced in the mid-20th century by TV game shows.

EXAMINATION ROOM, n.
Theatre.

EXAMINATION ROOM, PSYCHIATRIC, n.
Theatre of the absurd.

EXAMINATION ROOM, RADIOLOGICAL, n.
X-rated theatre.

EXAMINATION ROOM, SURGICAL, n.
Drive-in theatre.

FEVER, n.
Infection's way of announcing, 'Darling, I'm hoooome.'

FRIGIDITY, n.
The absence of sexual desire. In classical Freudian terms, frigidity is understood to be a displacement of the much more fundamental fear of biting into a crusty, egg-mayonnaise roll. More recent theorists have suggested that frigidity may result from family curses, too many Bergman movies, or just the bad luck of being in the wrong place at the wrong time.

GESTATION, n.
Pregnancy arising from a practical joke, such as putting a pin hole in a diaphragm.

HEALTH, n.
Condition in which the doctor is so incompetent he cannot identify the disease(s) at work. This diagnosis is a strong indication for changing doctors.

HIPPOCAMPUS, n.
Fat farm.

HIPPOCRATES, n;
The father of medicine. The mother is not known, but she is believed to have been a golf pro.

HYPERVENTILATE, v.
To breathe deeply and rapidly as an expression of anxiety. This tactic lowers the level of carbon dioxide in the blood, producing dizziness, numbness of the hand, tingling around the mouth, trembling of the limbs, and a rapid, faint heart beat. If you work at it, you can pass out. For a complete set of these and other exercises you can do in the lavatory at work, send £2 for our free booklet, 'Twenty Days to Feeling Funny.'

IATROGENIC, adj.
Referring to any disorder or disease arising as a complication of medical care; virtually unknown if you ask the BMA.

IDIOPATHIC, adj.
Referring to entities with origins that are unknown or cannot be explained, such as diseases like Lethal Midline Granuloma or punk rock songs like 'I'm Turning Japanese.'

IMPOTENCE, n.
Inability of the male to have intercourse the normal physiological maximum of once per night. Maybe twice. Might mean cancer. The appropriate response is understanding, kindness, and something to eat.

KINESIA, n.
See AKINESIA.

KNEECAP, n.
1. Form of persuasion unique to modern Irish politics.
2. A drink poured across the legs shortly before retiring to bed.

LABYRINTH, n.
1. Intricate communicating pathways of the inner ear.
2. The floor plan of any major hospital. Lost visitors are often used for organ transplants.

LANDOUZY-DEJERINE DISEASE, n.
Completely atrophy of the muscles of one side of the face. A cure for duplicity.

LAPAROTOMY, n.
Surgical procedure in which the abdomen is explored for an unknown source of disease; technique by which the doctor calls the hypochondriac's bluff.

LIPOPEXIA, n.
A medical term referring to the storage of fat. We suggest a basement cupboard protected from sunlight and moths.

MALPRACTICE, n.
According to your current doctor, medicine as practised by all of your doctors before him.

MAMMOPLASTY, n.
Cosmetic surgery of the breast; the triumph of hope over experience.

MORON, n.
Critic of *The Hypochondriac's Handbook*.

MOTHER, n.
A womb of one's own.

NAUSEA, n.
Sensation experienced while the body decides whether to throw up or just die.

NEISSERIA, n.
Ten genus of bacteria responsible for gonorrhea, known among doctors as the gift that never stops giving.

ONSET, n.
Beginning – usually, of the end.

OPTHALMOLOGIST, n.
Specialist who looks in your eyes while robbing you blind.

PALM, n.
Inner surface of the hand, subject to many disorders, notably *Palmar pruritus* – literally, itchy palms, a common problem among private doctors. This disease is responsive only to rapid and repeated injections of gold into tax shelters.

PENIS, n.
The male sexual organ. Vestigial with respect to its original function of grasping branches while swinging in trees, it now serves principally as a conversation piece, except in parts of northern England, where conversation does not exist.

PHLEGM, n.
Sputum or mucus; a medical term developed to trip up precocious children in spelling tests.

PHYSICAL THERAPY, n.
A massagenous ritual by which nubile young women remind critically ill patients that being bedridden isn't so bad after all.

PLACEBO, n.
See VITAMIN.

PLACENTA, n.
Afterbirth; biological proof that sequels never live up to the original.

POLYP, n.
Tumour on a stalk; the body's version of Land's End.

POUCH OF DOUGLAS, n.
A small pouch between the uterus and the rectum of

little use and less interest. However, considerable curiosity persists in the scientific community about just what Dr. Douglas was doing poking around in there.

PROCREATE, v.
To bring forth young; the opposite of recreate.

PROGNOSIS, n.
Doctor's best guess at how much time you have left.

PROSTATE, n.
Never order this in a Chinese restaurant.

PROTEIN, n.
Class of nitrogen-containing compounds once thought to be nutritionally important; now known to be useful primarily as a shampoo additive.

PTYALISM, n.
Excessive salivation, seen in rabies and pregnancy; one reason you should always keep a body of water between a pregnant woman and yourself.

PURULENT, adj.
Full of puss. Term developed to save doctors from embarrassing themselves by making indecent adjective out of the word 'pus,' A noble experiment in a lost cause.

QUACK, n.
Doctor who sticks obstinately by absurd theories that we do not entertain.

RABIES, n.
Viral inflammation of the brain contracted by kissing dogs on the lips.

REFERRAL, n.
An act whereby one doctor attests to the high temperature of a case and passes it on to another.

REMISSION, n.
Spontaneous abatement of a disease's symptoms occurring so unexpectedly that the doctors involved are unable to claim credit for it.

RHINERYNTER, n.
An elastic bag used for dilating the nostrils. Honest.

RIGA'S DISEASE, n.
A little ulcer under the tongue; can come from kissing doorknobs.

SCATOLOGY, n.
The study of faeces. No kidding.

SECOND OPINION, n.
Another throw of the medical dice.

SEX, n.
Behaviour related to reproduction. Currently, that is. In prehistoric times, sex was employed principally as a form of greeting between nomadic tribes. In 10,000 B.C., the handshake was invented in the region known as Basingstoke, Mesopotamia. Sexual intercourse as a form of greeting completely ceased, as the handshake conveyed friendliness without forcing one to get as sweaty. A world away, the Chinese were growing tired of reproduction by movable type, the compass, and gunpowder, all of which they had already invented. They applied the technique of sexual intercourse to proliferation. Soon other nations were forced to take up sex out of self-defence. And that's how we got into the mess we're in today.

SIDE EFFECT, n.
Pain in the flank that comes on with jogging.

SPHERESTHESIA, n.
A morbid sensation or dread of contact with a ball.
Prominent victims have included Geoff Boycott,
Buster Mottram and the entire Hereford football team.

SYPHILIS, n.
In Italy, The French Disease; in France, The Italian
Disease; in London's Soho, The Plague. If syphilis
didn't exist, Mary Whitehouse would have invented it.

TAENIOPHOBIA, n.
A morbid fear of becoming infected with tapeworms —
in our opinion a fear that is perfectly justified.

TESTOTERONE, n.
An Italian vitamin.

TOMOMANIA, n.
The abnormal desire to operate or to be operated upon.
There is an immediate electricity when a tomomaniac
surgeon and a similarly afflicted patient spot each
other across a crowded room. Till death do them part.

TRACHEOTOMY, n.
Means never having to say you're sorry.

TRICHINOSIS, n.
A pig's revenge.

TRUSS, n.
An elastic band designed to restrain abdominal
contents and prevent devastation of the countryside.

UNDINISM, n.
The awakening of sexual desire by running water.
Those afflicted with this preoccupation are easily
spotted by their ecstatic expressions at Niagra Falls.
Often accompanied by an abnormal fear of reservoirs.

VAGINA, n.
Aren't you a little old to be looking up words like this?

VEGETATIVE STATE, n.
Blunting of emotions and slowing of other intellectual functions seen in most heterosexual men upon confronting salads made with avocados, cottage cheese, or beetroot.

VITAMINS, n.
See PLACEBO.

VIRUS, n.
Agents causing all diseases doctors can't explain or cure with a pill.

The Book Of
ROYAL
LISTS

CRAIG BROWN & LESLEY CUNLIFFE

What should you serve the Royal Family if they drop in for dinner?
How does the Queen keep her Corgies content?
Which clergyman did Prince Charles throw into the fountain at Balmoral?
What are Princess Diana's favourite sweets?
Which television programmes does the Queen Mother like best?
How can you recognise a Royal racing pigeon?

The Royal Family is no ordinary family, and Royal Lists are not like ordinary lists. Here at last are the answers to all the questions that have intrigued dedicated Royal-watchers, loyal patriots, convinced monarchists and the millions of adoring fans around the world who follow every move of Britain's first family.

THE BOOK OF ROYAL LISTS is the most comprehensive collection of information ever assembled about the British Royal Family and their ancestors. Witty and informed, amusing but respectful, it surprises, charms and dazzles.

HUMOUR 0 7221 1934 8 £2.50

STRANGE THINGS

ROBERT K. G. TEMPLE

DID YOU KNOW THAT . . .

There may be two suns in the solar system!

Canaries lose a fifth of their brains in the winter – but get it all back in the spring!

The lesbian whiptail lizards of America clone their offspring!

There are planets in our galaxy which are 17% crystallized diamonds!

Some birds have a fear of flying!

STRANGE THINGS:

a bizarre, baffling and mind-boggling guide to the quirks of nature, including . . . heavy-breathing water lilies, sun-tanned eggs, irate embryos, perfumed moths, sensitive sponges, mathematical monkeys, over-sexed fruitflies and many other wonders.

SCIENCE   0 7221 8410 7   £1.50

TONIGHT
JOSEPHINE

and other undiscovered letters
Michael Green

IF . . .

Julius Caesar had gone for a picnic and left the Senate to have a stab at something else

Hitler had taken his ever-loving mother's advice about his friends (especially the fat one)

Archimedes' plumbing had got him into hot water

Napoleon had had more than wandering hand trouble

. . . History would have been very, very different!

Here at last are the letters which changed the world (or would have if they'd ever been written).

'Delightfully engaging . . . could prove even more popular than his huge successes *The Art of Coarse Rugby*, *The Art of Coarse Sailing*, etc.'
Sunday Express

HUMOUR   0 7221 4084 3   £1.25

LEONARD ROSSITER

THE LOWEST FORM OF WIT

Sarcasm is the lowest form of wit — no one is beneath using it — but it is also the most satisfying. There is no greater pleasure than pinning your squirming victim to the dinner-table with a carefully sharpened and coolly aimed insult or flooring him with a sudden and crippling kick beneath the belt.

Sarcasm requires deadly accuracy and perfect timing. It is the most skilful kind of unarmed combat and because no holds are barred it is also the most dangerous. THE LOWEST FORM OF WIT is a complete handbook for aspiring masters and mistresses of sarcasm compiled by Leonard Rossiter, a black belt of this vicious art. He tells you everything you need to know about sarcasm from its low-down role in history to specific advice on dealing with traffic wardens, bank managers, neighbours, foreigners and other despicable persons.

This is a treasury of biting jibes and stinging retorts which explores the lowest kind of wit in the highest kind of style.

HUMOUR   0 7221 7513 2   £1.50